RECENT ADVANCES IN VIRUS DIAGNOSIS

CURRENT TOPICS IN VETERINARY MEDICINE AND ANIMAL SCIENCE

RECENT ADVANCES IN VIRUS DIAGNOSIS

A Seminar in the CEC Programme of Co-ordination of Research on Animal Pathology, held at the Veterinary Research Laboratories, Belfast, Northern Ireland, September 22–23, 1983

Sponsored by the Commission of the European Communities, Directorate-General for Agriculture, Co-ordination of Agricultural Research

Edited by

M.S. McNulty and J.B. McFerran
Veterinary Research Laboratories, Belfast
Northern Ireland

1984 **MARTINUS NIJHOFF PUBLISHERS**
a member of the KLUWER ACADEMIC PUBLISHERS GROUP
BOSTON / THE HAGUE / DORDRECHT / LANCASTER
for
THE COMMISSION OF THE EUROPEAN COMMUNITIES

Distributors

for the United States and Canada: Kluwer Academic Publishers, 190 Old Derby Street, Hingham, MA 02043, USA
for the UK and Ireland: Kluwer Academic Publishers, MTP Press Limited, Falcon House, Queen Square, Lancaster LA1 1RN, England
for all other countries: Kluwer Academic Publishers Group, Distribution Center, P.O. Box 322, 3300 AH Dordrecht, The Netherlands

Library of Congress Catalog Card Number   84-14889

ISBN-13:978-94-009-6041-1   e-ISBN-13:978-94-009-6039-8
DOI: 10.1007/978-94-009-6039-8
EUR 8917 EN

Book information

Publication arranged by: Commission of the European Communities, Directorate-General Information Market and Innovation, Luxembourg

Copyright/legal notice

Preface

The traditional approach to diagnosis of virus infections by isolation of the causative virus is usually both slow and expensive. More recently, the emphasis has been on the direct detection of viruses or viral antigens in clinical specimens. This can be done using established techniques such as immunofluorescence or electron microscopy, or by newly developed biochemical methods. The purpose of this meeting was to review these and other developments in the laboratory diagnosis of virus infections.

We would like to thank all those who contributed to the success of this meeting. In particular, we are grateful to the CEC for financial sponsorship, to Professor C. Dow, Director of the Veterinary Research Laboratories, for help in organising the meeting, and to Miss B. Hamilton for her excellent typing of the manuscripts.

M S McNulty

J B McFerran

CONTENTS

VIII

VIRAL DIAGNOSIS BY IMMUNOFLUORESCENCE

P.S. Gardner

Division of Microbiological Reagents and Quality Control
Central Public Health Laboratory
175 Colindale Avenue
London, NW9 5HT

ABSTRACT

The main use of immunofluorescence in both human and veterinary virology should be for the rapid detection of antigen at site of lesion. For human disease WHO has strongly recommended immunofluorescence for rapid diagnosis of respiratory infection by detecting virus in nasopharyngeal secretions, and in the absence of an electron microscope for the investigation of skin and eye scrapings and brain biopsies. The principle of the technique and its methodology are briefly outlined and the use of conventional, egg-derived and monoclonal antibodies discussed. Some further advantages of the immunofluorescence technique are mentioned such as the investigation of outbreaks of respiratory disease in an animal house, the detection of antigen in secretions after infectivity of virus is lost, investigation of post-mortem specimens, control of cross-infection and diagnosis of infection at a distance from the virus laboratory. The major criticism of immunofluorescence is its labour intensiveness, which is balanced by its increased sensitivity and so far comparisons with alternative techniques such as ELISA have confirmed this increased sensitivity. Conjugated-staphylococcal protein A would appear to have no part in this technology as discussed and little information is available on the use of biotin-avidin as a detection system. Automation of reading fluorescence has been attempted by use of time-resolved fluoroimmunoassay, but it is too early to judge whether this technique is sufficiently practical, reproducible and economic for universal use.

IMMUNOFLUORESCENCE

In human medicine, and it should be no different in veterinary medicine, viral diagnosis to be meaningful, has to be rapid, which means at a time when that diagnosis can influence management of the patient or sick animal, or influence the progress of infection in a community or a herd.

Appropriately, immunofluorescence has been put first on this programme, perhaps by chance, or, perhaps because it does represent the forerunner of practical rapid virus diagnostic procedures from which most of the other modern techniques have been developed. Less universally acceptable is the concept that immunofluorescence is the most rapid of techniques available. For example, in the case of rotavirus infections, from source to answer can be measured in minutes by using electron microscopy. Therefore, immunofluorescence must be looked at within the context of what its present diagnostic potential is, how it may develop in the future and its present role among the current rapid diagnostic methods, for no single diagnostic method can be applied to all clinical situations.

The principle upon which immunofluorescence has been based is illustrated in Fig. 1 where a fluorochrome dye such as fluorescein isothiocyanate has been excited by light of certain wavelengths and in reverting to

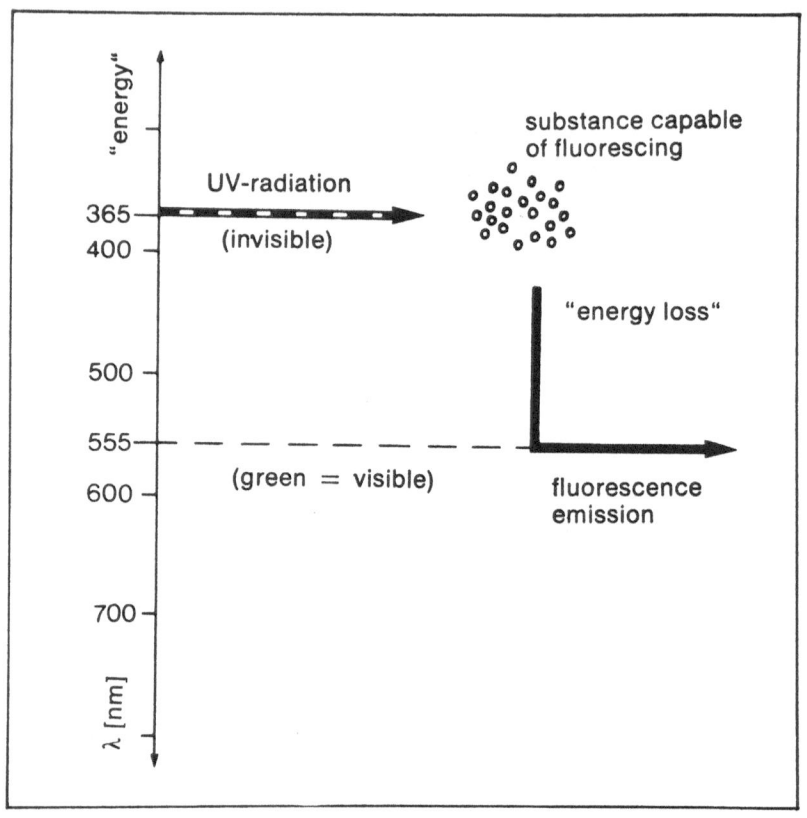

Fig. 1   Diagramatic illustration of excitation of fluorochrome dye and its reversion to its resting state.

its original resting state emits light of longer wavelengths than that which stimulated it.

Fluorochromes absorb light preferentially and the wavelength of maximum absorption for excitation of fluorescein isothiocyanate is 490 nm and the maximum wavelength for emission is 517 nm in the green part of the spectrum (Fig. 2). Ideally fluorescein should be irradiated at the wavelength of maximum absorption, but as this is so close to maximum emission problems appear with ordinary light filtration systems and this led to the

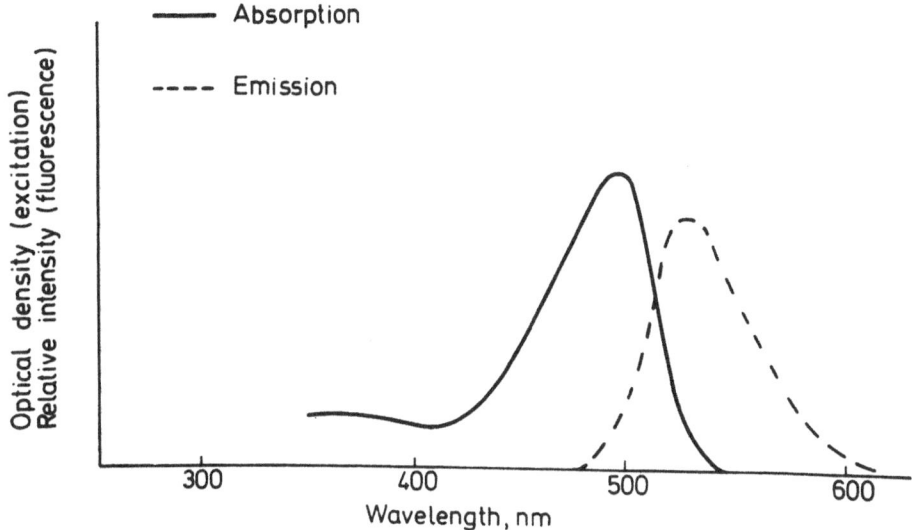

Fig. 2   The wavelengths of maximum absorption and emission for fluorescein isothiocyanate.

introduction of interference filters which can transmit light up to 490 nm with a sharp cut-off at 500 nm (Fig. 3); Fig. 4 shows the appropriate barrier filter for this system. This basically is the principle behind fluorescence microscopy.

In practice, diagnosis by immunofluorescence can be used as either a direct or as an indirect test. The indirect test is useful when a large number of different antigens are being sought and a common antispecies globulin can be used. It also produces a brighter picture as more fluorescein molecules are involved. The direct test is obviously a quicker technique as it has one stage less and it is appropriate where one is only looking for a single antigen.

Rapid diagnosis by immunofluorescence depends on identifying the causal agent in clinical material taken from the patient. This technique is now mainly applied to the diagnosis of respiratory infections. Respiratory secretions are collected by suction through a fine catheter. The aim of the procedure is to obtain intact cells. Secretions are diluted in phosphate buffered saline, centrifuged at 1,000 rpm, the cells are resuspended in a small amount of phosphate buffered saline and placed on prepared teflon coated slides, dried in air and fixed in acetone at 4°C for 10 minutes.

4

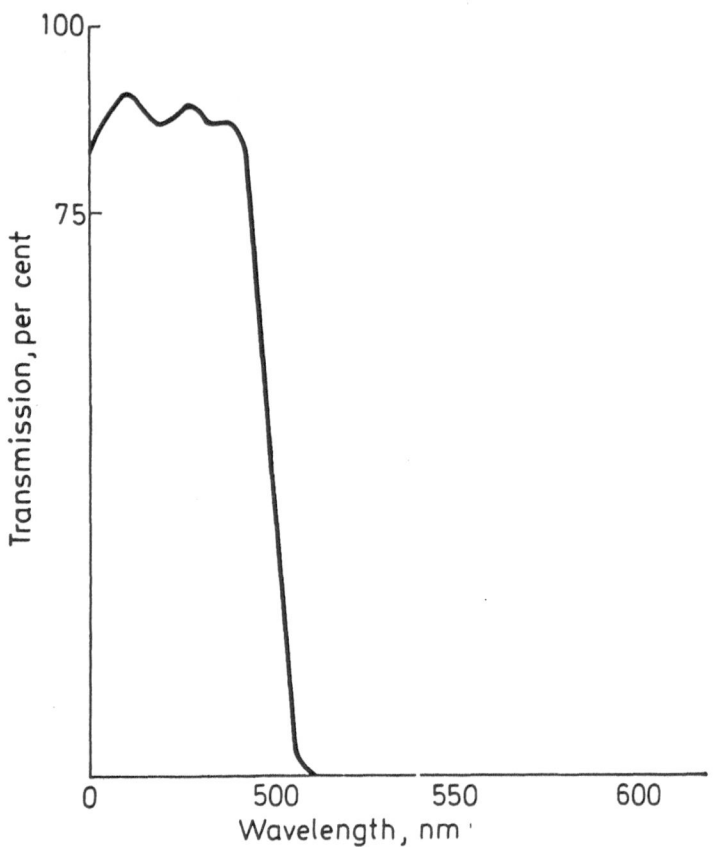

Fig. 3   The interference filter for transmitting light up to 490 nm.

Staining consists of putting on the appropriate specific virus antiserum
for 30 mins at 37°C, washing for 30 mins in phosphate buffered saline, 30
mins in antispecies conjugate at 37°C, rewashing for 30 mins in buffer with
a final rinse in distilled water for 1 min to prevent crystal formation.
The slide is then dried in air and examined in blue light under oil immer-
sion, there being no need to use a coverslip.

The taking of the specimens, their preparation and staining have been
fully described elsewhere (Gardner and McQuillin, 1980). All viral antigens
occurring in secretions can be detected by immunofluorescence. Fig. 5 and
Fig. 6 show two examples of viruses which cause severe illness in both the
human infant and calf viz. respiratory syncytial virus and parainfluenza

virus type 3.

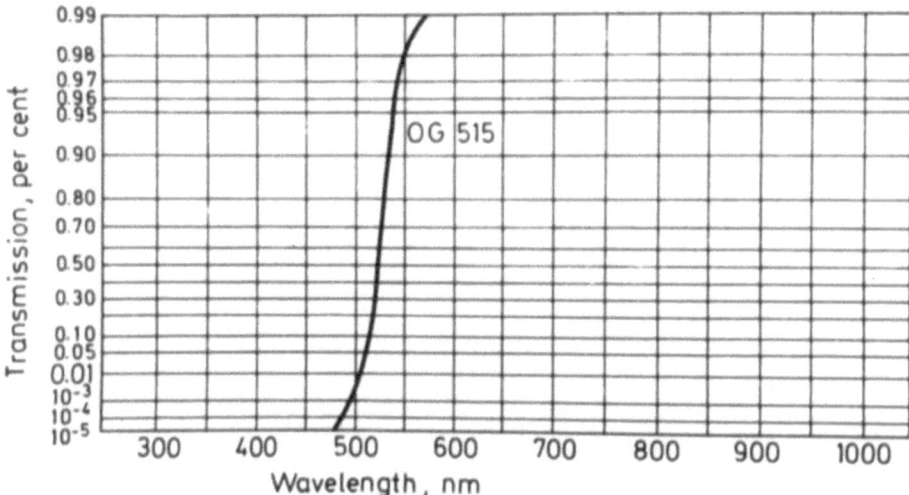

Fig. 4 The appropriate barrier filter for use with interference filter illustrated in Fig. 3.

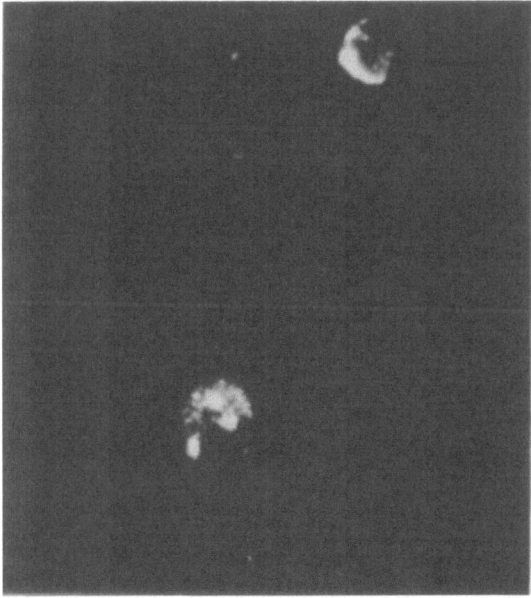

Fig. 5 Cells in nasopharyngeal secretions containing RS virus antigen of infant with bronchiolitis.

6

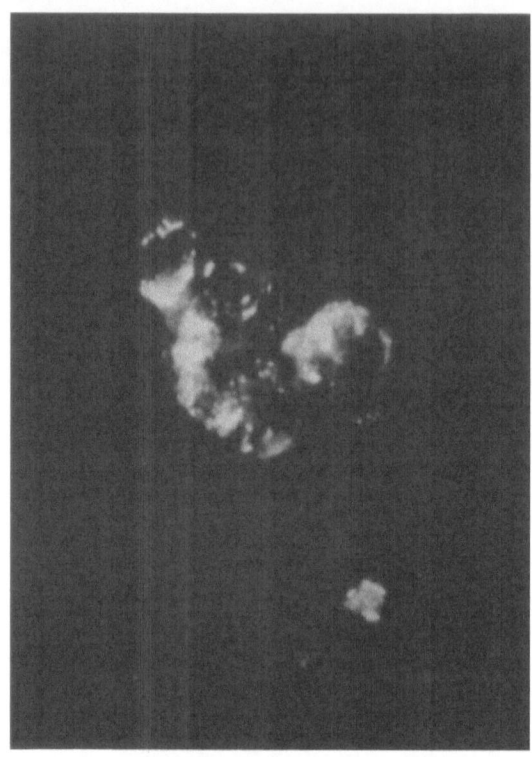

Fig. 6   Cells in nasopharyngeal secretions containing parainfluenza
virus type 3 antigen in a child with croup.

The antisera used in the above systems were bovine, which had commercial advantages in being derived from large animals with serum available
in large quantities. Furthermore, bovines are natural hosts of both these
organisms so titres were high and relatively little purification was necessary.

However, a few virus antisera were difficult to prepare in bovines
such as adenovirus group, influenza B and parainfluenza virus type 1. Rather
than use the uneconomic system of the rabbit a new method was attempted by
Dr June D Almeida at Wellcome Research Laboratories of inoculating laying
hens with the appropriate virus and harvesting the yolk sac for specific
egg anti-globulins. This has been highly successful and in conjunction
with Division of Microbiological Reagents and Quality Control at Colindale,
quality-assessed highly-specific reagents have been produced which have
replaced some of the current antisera with a battery of egg derived ones
(Table 1) (Gardner and Kaye, 1982).

TABLE 1   Antisera available for use in the fluorescent antibody technique.

Bovine	"Egg"	Rabbit (Obsolete)	To be achieved
Respiratory syncytial virus	Influenza A	Influenza B	Parainfluenza 2
Influenza A	Influenza B	Parainfluenza 1	Mumps
Parainfluenza 3	Parainfluenza 1	Adenovirus group	
Measles	Parainfluenza 3		
	Adenovirus group		

A further new development in antibody production has been the use of monoclonal antibodies and the author's Department has produced a number of monoclonal antibodies to adenovirus types 3 and 5 which are type, subtype and group specific. The group specific ones are of special interest as they could replace conventional antisera if they were capable of detecting the appropriate epitopes of all wild adenovirus strains (Russell et al., 1981). This aspect is now being assessed. The appearance of the infected cells in secretions using the three different antibodies is identical ie rabbit, egg globulin and monoclonal.

A further example of the effectiveness of immunofluorescence in diagnosis may be seen in Fig. 7 which is an impression smear of a lung of a marmoset who among others died of a severe respiratory infection in a research animal house. This was shown conclusively by immunofluorescence to have been an outbreak of parainfluenza virus type 1. Masses of parainfluenza virus-like particles were found by electron microscopy (Almeida, 1984). Antisera from convalescent marmosets all showed antibodies to parainfluenza virus type 1, but those from a colony of marmosets which had been kept well separated from the infected ones showed no antibody at all.

Among other advantages of the fluorescence antibody technique is the ability to detect antigen after the infectivity of the secretion is lost, and infected cells in the convalescent phase of the illness show a hazy fluorescent appearance due to a coating of patient's own antibody. This appearance therefore explains why virus is difficult to isolate at this stage and why immunofluorescence is more sensitive (Gardner and McQuillin, 1978).

There are many other advantages of using immunofluorescence for rapid virus diagnosis, among which are the control and prevention of ward

8

infections (Gardner et al., 1973).

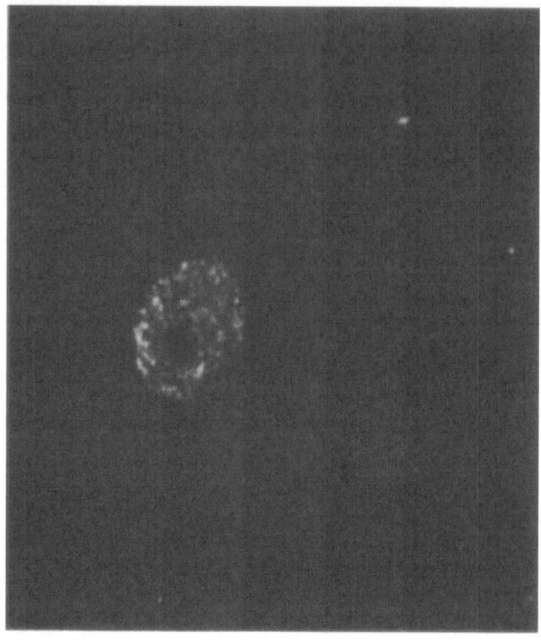

Fig. 7   Impression smear of parainfluenza virus type 1 infected cell of a lung of a marmoset.

If slides are prepared and fixed they may be sent long distances to be examined by a virus laboratory; this procedure could be of great advantage in developing countries and in the UK an effective postal diagnostic service was run for Cumbria from a Newcastle laboratory (Downham et al., 1974).

It is also an ideal method for examining autopsy material of those who have died of respiratory infections and the causal viral agent can be demonstrated at the site of damage. Fig. 8 shows an impression smear of a lung from a human infant who died of bronchiolitis caused by respiratory syncytial virus (Downham et al., 1975).

WHO in its various memoranda, monographs and meetings has quite unequivocally decided that at this moment in time immunofluorescence is the method of choice for the examination of respiratory specimens for virus infections (Memorandum, WHO Bulletin, 1977; Memorandum, WHO Bulletin, 1978). So much so that it has organised the training of staff in teaching meetings held all over the world, and by assessing the results and supplying reagents of impeccable quality has brought virus diagnosis to parts of the world that had never previously had this facility.

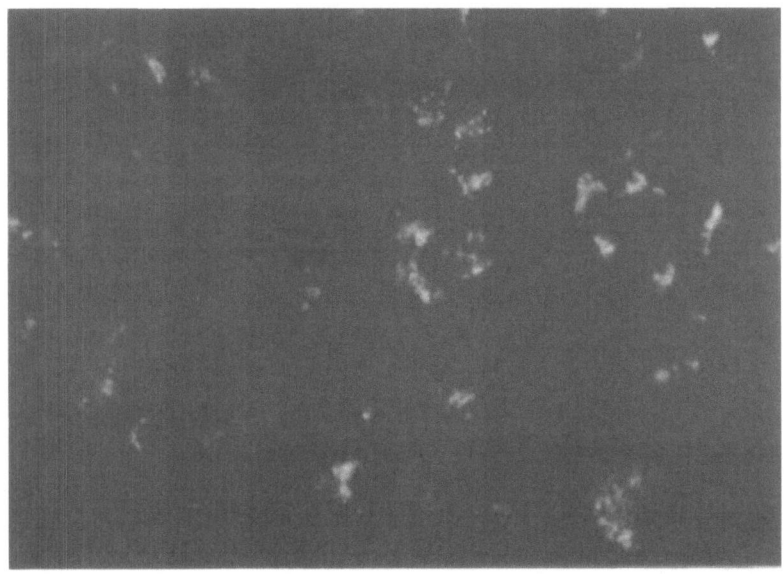

Fig. 8   Impression smear of RS virus infected lung cells of an infant who died of bronchiolitis.

WHO and even the most fervent proponents of immunofluorescence recognise certain disadvantages in the method in the large labour intensiveness of the work involved, the need for highly trained staff and in the long run one is making a personal professional judgement not an automated machine print-out decision. It is probably this latter factor which gives immunofluorescence the edge in sensitivity and accuracy. WHO has agreed that other methods such as ELISA should be examined in detail to see if their smaller labour intensiveness could be exploited and accordingly a trial was mounted between the author's Department and that of Dr Grandien of the National Bacteriological Laboratory, Stockholm who is a proponent of ELISA as well as immunofluorescence. Table 2 summarises the results of this trial. Secretions were prepared by ward staff and a duplicate secretion as a slide sent to the author's laboratory. At the time that the immunofluorescence tests were performed on these slides the ELISA results were unknown.

There is no doubt of the decreased sensitivity of ELISA which is understandable since one only needs to observe a single positive cell to know when the specimen is positive by immunofluorescence. Though fluorescence was not routinely performed by Dr Grandien, by chance she confirmed by

TABLE 2   Comparison of results by the fluorescent antibody technique
and ELISA on nasopharyngeal secretions.

	Influenza A	Parainfluenza 3	RSV	Negatives	Total
Division of Microbiological Reagents and Quality Control, Colindale		Immunofluorescence results			
	15	2	18	38	73
National Bacteriological Laboratory, Stockholm		ELISA results			
	14	2	14	43	73

immunofluorescence four of the five failures by ELISA. Similar trials in
Stockholm, Copenhagen and elsewhere have repeatedly confirmed this small
but significant difference in sensitivity between ELISA and immunofluorescence. There is also great truth in the cliche "that seeing is believing"
and the specificity of the reaction can be controlled by eye by seeing the
right coloured apple-green fluorescence and by seeing it intracellularly in
the right type of cell and with the right distribution within that cell.

A word about non-respiratory specimens. WHO felt that the electron
microscope was the method of choice for the examination of specimens taken
from skin and eye scrapings, but in the event of laboratories not having an
electron microscope, which still occurs from time to time, then immunofluorescence would be a good second choice.

It might be profitable to speculate as to how immunofluorescence can
be improved further in sensitivity and in becoming less labour intensive.
Since the introduction of immunofluorescence for rapid virus diagnosis, two
methods of improving the conjugates and increasing the sensitivity have
been advocated, neither have been adapted for the detection of viral antigens in clinical material.

The first is the use of staphylococcal protein A. This protein binds
to the Fc portion of many immunoglobulins but not to the antigen-binding
Fab fragment. In theory one could use a fluorescein-labelled staphylococcal
protein A complex as the indicator of any antigen-antibody reaction. Staphylococcal protein A has several advantages over antiglobulins as illustrated
in Table 3 but its disadvantages probably outweigh these.

TABLE 3   Advantages and disadvantages of Staphylococcal Protein A.

Advantages over antiglobulin

1. It is available in pure form
2. Is a stable molecule under a variety of conditions
3. It reacts with the immunoglobulins of most mammalian species
4. It can be conjugated with a number of marker molecules with little or no loss of immunoglobulin-binding activity
5. It exhibits low nonspecific binding to materials and reagents
6. It is not bound by Fc receptors present on herpesviruses and herpesvirus-infected cells.

Disadvantages over antiglobulin

1. It does not detect IgG_3, IgM, IgA
2. It may have a lower affinity than antiglobulins
3. It reacts poorly with certain species especially avian

Antiglobulins detect certain immunoglobulins which protein A will not, such as IgG_3, IgM and IgA. A specific antiglobulin of particular high affinity may provide greater sensitivity than protein A. Most important is the varying reaction with immunoglobulins of various species. Reaction is poor with goat and sheep immunoglobulin and non-existent with avian. The last is especially important since the modern trend towards the use of the easy method of production of specific globulins in eggs. The subject has been reviewed by Richman (1983).

A similar situation arises with the avidin-biotin system. There is a high affinity between the glycoprotein avidin and the vitamin biotin. In its hydroxysuccinimide form biotin binds to antibodies. Avidin can be labelled with fluorescein and a system either in a simple or an enchancing bridge form as shown in Fig. 9 can be devised. Theoretically the bridge form could give an increased sensitivity. However no virologists appear to have used this system for antigen detection to date though the potential is there.

The basic problem with immunofluorescence is the inability up to now to automate its reading as the human eye has been necessary to distinguish background nonspecific fluorescence from specific intracellular fluorescence. A new principle has been developed by Halonen and his colleagues (1983) in Turku known as time-resolved fluoroimmunoassay. Very briefly, it

12

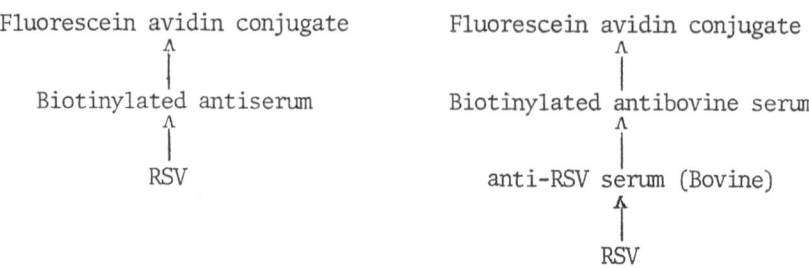

Fig. 9   A simple and bridge form of the Avidin-Biotin system.

depends on having a fluorescent probe with a long lifetime, excited by a
short light pulse and specific fluorescence is measured after a selected
delay time. During the delay time, background fluorescence which has a
short decay is eliminated and specific fluorescence is detected. The rare
earth metal europium has a long decay time 100 - 1000 us and also when conjugated has a large difference between excitation and emission wavelengths
which results in a further reduction in background noise. The test is
similar to any other assay (Fig. 10). The specimens are read in a single-
photon counting fluorometer equipped with a xenon flash lamp. The

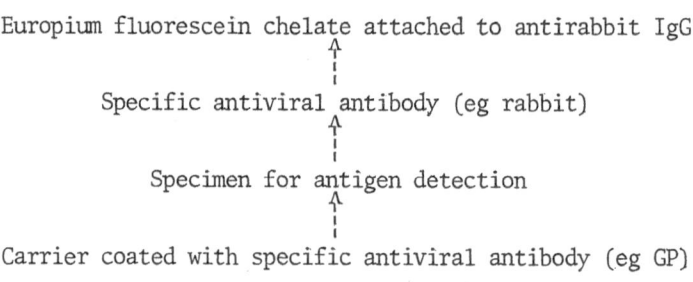

Fig. 10   The stages of time-resolved fluoroimmunoassay.

excitation wavelength is 340 nm and the length of excitation pulse is 1 μs.
After delay of 400 μs single photon emission is counted for 500 μs at 613 nm.
After a further delay of 100 μs a new cycle begins. The cycle is repeated
1000 times in overall counting time of 1 second. The Turku workers are apparently the only ones who have used this diagnostically to date and their
results compare very favourably with RIA and conventional fluorescence. Is
this the shape of things to come or a flash in the dark representing a
piece of exciting new technology? Will the sophisticated equipment for

reading become sufficiently cheap as to constitute a piece of routine equipment or will it remain in the realms of the fantastic never travelling beyond research laboratories? As a first stage the results of Turku must be confirmed elsewhere and compared with conventional techniques.

When rapid diagnosis started it revolved round the fluorescent antibody technique and electron microscopy. The scientist enjoyed great personal satisfaction as with his own eyes he was making a decision and a diagnosis, and as an additional bonus he could admire the beauty of his work (Fig. 11). We as a breed are now being replaced by the scientist who gets

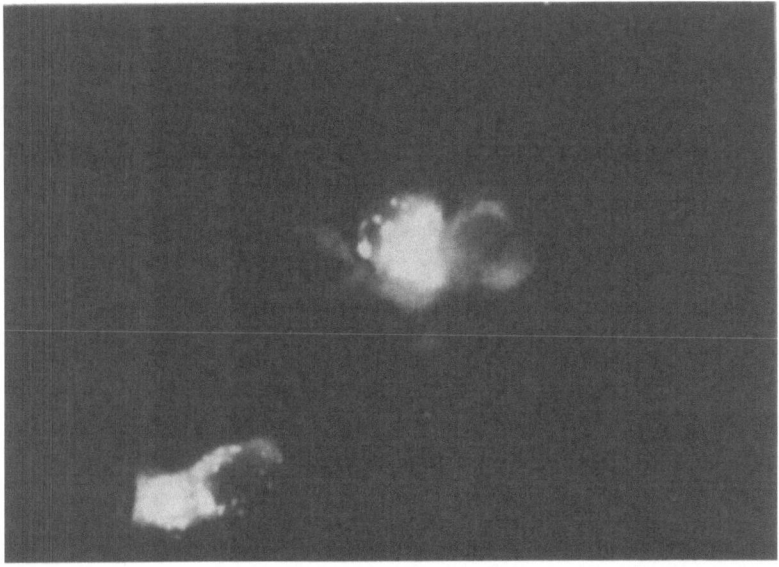

Fig. 11   Cells of nasopharyngeal secretions containing parainfluenza virus type 2 from a child with severe croup.

his kicks from the excitement of reading endless reams of ticker-tape under the cry of all that can be done on a large scale is beautiful. We really need to complete the circle and ask ourselves the questions, are all the thousands upon thousands of investigations that are being done really necessary, does every one of these tests have a patient benefit and can we really afford the sophistication that is being forced on us when simpler techniques would still supply all the wants of routine diagnosis?

REFERENCES

Almeida, J.D. 1984. Electron microscopy. Recent Advances in Virus Diagnosis, (this volume).

14

Downham, M.A.P.S., Elderkin, F.M., Platt, J.W., McQuillin, J. and Gardner, P.S. 1974. Rapid Virus Diagnosis in Paediatric Units by a Postal Service: Respiratory syncytial virus infection in Cumberland. Arch. Dis. in Childhood, 49, 467-471.

Downham, M.A.P.S., Gardner, P.S., McQuillin, J. and Ferris, J.A.J. 1975. Role of respiratory viruses in childhood mortality. Brit. Med. J., 1, 235-239.

Gardner, P.S., Court, S.D.M., Brocklebank, J.T., Downham, M.A.P.S. and Weightman, D. 1973. Virus Cross-infection in Paediatric Wards. Brit. Med. J., 2, 571-575.

Gardner, P.S. and McQuillin, J. 1978. The coating of R.S. virus infected cells in the respiratory tract by immunoglobulins. J. Med. Virol., 2, 77-87.

Gardner, P.S. and McQuillin, J. 1980. Rapid Virus Diagnosis. Application of immunofluorescence. 2nd Edition. (Butterworths, London).

Gardner, P.S. and Kaye, S. 1982. Egg globulins in rapid virus diagnosis. J. Virol. Methods, 4, 257-262.

Halonen, P., Meurman, O., Lovgren, T., Hemmila, I. and Soini, E. 1983. Current topics in Microbiology and Immunology, Vol. 104. New Developments in Diagnostic Virology. Detection of viral antigens by time-resolved fluoroimmunoassay (Ed. Peter A. Bachmann). (Springer-Verlag, Berlin, Heidelberg). pp. 133-146.

Memorandum. 1977. Laboratory techniques for rapid diagnosis of viral infections. Bulletin of the World Health Organization, 55, 33-37.

Memorandum. 1978. Progress in the rapid diagnosis of viral infections. Bulletin of the World Health Organization, 56, 241-244.

Richman, D.D. 1983. Current topics in Microbiology and Immunology, Vol. 104. New Developments in Diagnostic Virology. The use of staphylococcal Protein A in diagnostic virology. (Ed. Peter A. Bachmann). pp. 159-176.

Russell, W.C., Patel, G., Precious, B., Sharp, I. and Gardner, P.S. 1981. Monoclonal antibodies against Adenovirus Type 5; Preparation and preliminary characterisation. J. Gen. Virol., 56, 393-408.

APPLICATIONS OF IMMUNOFLUORESCENCE IN VETERINARY VIRAL DIAGNOSIS

M.S. McNulty and G.M. Allan

Veterinary Research Laboratories
Stormont, Belfast BT4 3SD
Northern Ireland

ABSTRACT

This paper describes some applications of immunofluorescence in the laboratory diagnosis of veterinary virus infections. These include (1) the direct examination of clinical material for virus antigens, a procedure particularly useful for rapid diagnosis of Aujeszky's disease and bovine respiratory disease (2) the recognition of the growth of 'difficult' and/or non-cytopathogenic viruses eg avian infectious bronchitis virus in eggs and BVD virus and rotaviruses in cell cultures (3) the detection of viral antibodies by indirect immunofluorescence and (4) the recognition of new viruses eg an entero-like virus associated with runting in broiler chickens.

INTRODUCTION

This paper describes the principle applications of immunofluorescence in virus diagnosis in this laboratory. These fall into 4 main categories (a) direct examination of clinical material for virus antigens, (b) recognition of the growth of 'difficult' and/or non-cytopathogenic viruses in various culture systems, (c) detection of viral antibodies by indirect immunofluorescence and (d) recognition of new viruses.

MATERIALS AND METHODS

Conjugation of antisera

Antisera for direct immunofluorescence were conjugated with fluorescein isothiocyanate isomer 1 (FITC) (Sigma Chemical Company Ltd., London).

Ten ml amounts of sera were cooled in an ice bath and the globulin precipitated by slow addition of cold, saturated ammonium sulphate to a final concentration of 50% for mammalian antisera and 33% for avian antisera. The mixture was stirred for 15 mins and centrifuged for 10 mins at $4^{o}C$ at 4,000 g. The supernatants were discarded and the precipitated globulins resuspended in 10 ml 33% or 50% saturated ammonium sulphate solution in 0.15 M saline. These were centrifuged as before, the supernatants discarded and the precipitates resuspended in 10 ml 0.15 M saline. These solutions were dialysed against 100 volumes of 0.15 M saline for 2 days at $4^{o}C$. Following dialysis, the globulin solutions were centrifuged at 3,000 g for 10 mins and the total protein content estimated using a UV spectrophotometer at 280 nm (O.D. 1.0 = 1.0 mg protein/ml). FITC was added to the globulin solutions at a ratio of 3.5 mg FITC to 100 mg protein. The fluorescein powder was dissolved in 1.5 ml (15% total volume) of carbonate-bicarbonate buffer, pH 9.0 (3.7 g sodium bicarbonate and 0.6 g sodium carbonate in 100 ml water) and added slowly to the chilled globulins. The mixture was incubated at $4^{o}C$ for 18 hours with gentle stirring.

Six g Sephadex G25 was taken for each 10 ml labelled serum and swollen in phosphate-buffered saline (0.01 M phosphate, 0.15 NaCl, pH 7.2) (PBS). A column was poured with the Sephadex and the labelled serum added and eluted with PBS. The first peak was collected.

One g DEAE-cellulose was taken for each ml of conjugate and equilibrated in PBS. A column was poured, the labelled globulin was added and eluted with PBS. All the elutate which was green in colour was collected in small aliquots and tested for potency and specificity. The positive fractions were pooled, dispensed in 1 ml amounts and stored at $-70^{o}C$.

Absorption of conjugated antisera

All conjugates used for direct immunofluorescence were absorbed with tissue homogenates. In general, homogenates used for absorption were homologous with the tissue being examined and all conjugates were also absorbed with homogenised bovine lymph nodes. Material for homogenates was taken from animals which were demonstrated to be free of the virus under test and processed in the following manner. The tissue was washed in PBS, cut into small pieces and washed in PBS until free of blood. The tissue fragments were homogenised in an equal volume of PBS, frozen at $-70^{o}C$, thawed and centrifuged at 3,000 g for 20 mins. The cell deposit was resuspended in PBS and centrifuged as before. This was repeated until the supernatant was clear. After the final centrifugation the supernatant was decanted and the homogenised tissue deposit resuspended in a small volume of PBS to make a workable slurry. This was dispensed in 10 ml amounts and stored at $-20^{o}C$. For absorption, equal volumes of homogenate and conjugate were mixed for 24 hours at $4^{o}C$. The mixture was centrifuged at 5,000 g for 30 mins at $4^{o}C$ and the supernatant harvested. The absorption procedure was repeated and the final supernatant fluid passed through a 0.45 μ Millipore filter, dispensed in 1 ml amounts and frozen at $-70^{o}C$.

Procedures for preparation and immunofluorescent staining of tissues

Samples of nasal mucus were collected using a portable suction apparatus and shaken with glass beads in 10 ml amounts of PBS. They were decanted and centrifuged at 2,000 g for 10 mins and the supernatant discarded. The cell pellets were resuspended in 1 ml PBS and smears made on clean, degreased microscope slides. These were air dried at room temperature and fixed in acetone for 10 mins at room temperature (McNulty et al., 1983).

Impression smears from necropsy material were made as soon after death as possible and a number of different sites were taken from the tissues under test. These tissues were cut using a sterile scalpel blade and the clean freshly cut surfaces used to make the smears on degreased, glass microscope slides. Smears were dried and fixed in acetone as above.

Tissues for cryostat sections were placed in isopentane, chilled in a liquid nitrogen bath, transferred to a freezing cryostat and sections 4 μ thick cut. These were fixed in acetone for 30 mins at -20°C.

Cell cultures for immunofluorescence were grown on coverslips and fixed in acetone for 10 mins at room temperature.

Following fixation, tissues were stained for 1 hour at 37°C with FITC conjugates, washed in several changes of PBS for at least 30 mins, mounted in buffered glycerol, and examined using incident ultra-violet illumination.

Fluorescent microscope

All instrumentation was supplied by E Leitz (Instruments) Ltd., 48 Park Street, Luton. This comprised the following:

1. Ortholux 2 microscope stand.
2. Pleomopak 2.2 fluorescence illuminator.
3. Filter block 12-T-Auramine, FITC, FDA.
4. Stabilised starter unit XBO75/HBO100.
5. Lamphouse 100Z with HBO100 mercury vapour burner.
6. Fluorite oil X40/1.30 objective.
7. Periplan GF X10 eyepieces.
8. Supression filters. EGG455-1 EGG4751.

RESULTS AND DISCUSSION

Direct examination of clinical material

Direct immunofluorescent examination of clinical material has been more widely used in medical (Gardner and McQuillin, 1980) than veterinary virology. Its main advantage is speed. It avoids the necessity of isolating

the virus before identifying it, and combines, in one step, the dual ob-
jectives of virus detection and identification. The main problem with immunofluorescence is that interpretation of staining is sometimes rather
subjective and calls for considerable experience.

Direct immunofluorescence can be carried out on impression smears of
various tissues made on glass microscope slides or on cryostat sections.
The latter method has traditionally been the more widely used. Results
with cryostat sections are generally easier to interpret as the pattern of
staining and the precise location of fluorescing cells within a piece of
tissue can usually be established. Obviously, however, staining of impression smears is quicker and less laborious. A practical approach is to
examine material first by impression smears and to confirm positives and
doubtfuls by cryostat sections. Whatever method is used, a specific, high
titre primary antiserum is essential. Antisera which give little or no non-
specific staining with cultured cells may produce some non-specific staining with clinical material, particularly if large numbers of inflammatory
cells are present. This non-specific staining can usually be removed by
absorption with tissue homogenates. Because most commercially available
FITC-labelled antispecies immunoglobulins produce non-specific staining with
clinical material, we prefer to use the direct rather than the indirect
method of immunofluorescent staining.

Virus infections for which direct immunofluorescence is routinely used
for diagnosis in this laboratory are listed in Table I.

TABLE 1   Routine applications of direct immunofluorescence on
clinical material at Stormont.

Species	Specimens	Viruses
Bovine	(Nasal mucus (Lung* ((((Foetal tissues*	(Respiratory syncytial (Parainfluenza type 3 (Corona (BVD (IBR BVD
Porcine	(Brain, pharynx (Foetal tissue*	Aujeszky's disease Parvo
Fowl	(Bursa ((Trachea*	IBD (ILT (ND

* Cryostat sections preferable

Immunofluorescence has proved particularly useful for rapid diagnosis
of Aujeszky's disease in pigs (Fig. 1). Allan et al. (1984a) compared the

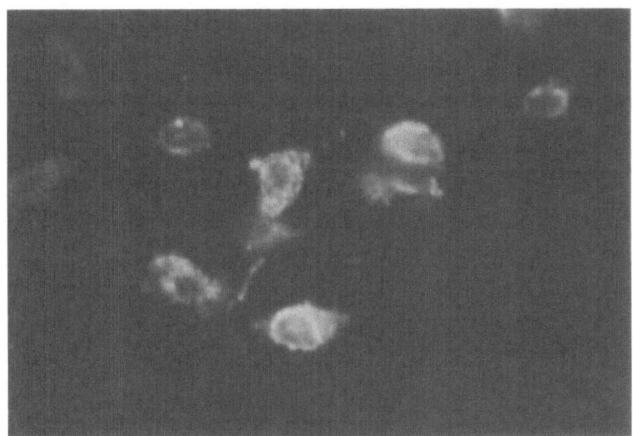

Fig. 1   Aujeszky's disease virus antigens in brain smear of young
pig which died with nervous signs.

sensitivity of immunofluorescence and virus isolation for detecting
Aujeszky's disease virus in experimentally infected pigs. Virus isolation
from pharynx was more successful than from brain specimens, reflecting the
higher titres of virus in the pharynx. Immunofluorescent staining of
pharyngeal impression smears was slightly more sensitive than virus isolation from pharynx in that immunofluorescence remained positive when circulating antibody prevented virus isolation. In contrast, immunofluorescent staining of impression smears of anterior and mid-cerebrum and medulla
oblongata was slightly less sensitive than virus isolation from the same
material. With 166 specimens of brain and pharynx from 78 suspected field
cases of Aujeszky's disease, there was 98% agreement between the results
obtained by virus isolation and immunofluorescent staining of pharyngeal
and brain impression smears. Apart from its speed and sensitivity, immunofluorescence has the advantage that it can still detect virus antigen in
material in which virus infectivity has been inactivated by post-mortem
autolysis.

Another useful application for direct immunofluorescent staining of
clinical material has been in the diagnosis of bovine respiratory disease,
particularly indoor calf pneumonia. The technique is particularly suitable
here because some of the viruses involved eg respiratory syncytial virus
(RSV) and coronavirus, are extremely difficult to isolate in cell cultures.

Furthermore, most isolates of bovine virus diarrhoea/mucosal disease (BVD) virus are non-cytopathogenic and immunofluorescent staining of infected cell cultures is necessary to demonstrate these. Mixed virus infections are sometimes associated with indoor calf pneumonia. These are easier to detect by direct immunofluorescence than by virus isolation. When virus isolation is used, slow growing viruses are usually eclipsed by rapidly growing viruses and may be missed. Epithelial cells present in samples of nasal mucus are examined for viral antigens by staining with a battery of conjugated antisera (McNulty et al., 1983). This works well with all the viruses listed in Table 1 (Fig. 2), except for BVD virus, where the low

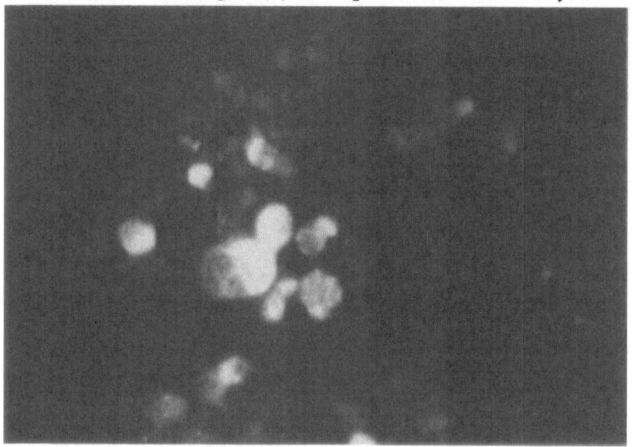

Fig. 2   Respiratory syncytial virus antigens in epithelial cells from nasal mucus of a calf with respiratory disease.

concentration of viral antigen and the diffuse pattern of staining can make interpretation very difficult. Impression smears and cryostat sections of lung tissue (Fig. 3) can be examined when necropsy material is available. In a study of calves experimentally infected with RSV, the results of immunofluorescent staining of lung impression smears were in complete agreement with those obtained using cryostat sections (McNulty et al., 1983).

Direct immunofluorescence on clinical specimens also has applications in avian diagnostic virology. Diagnosis of infectious bursal disease (IBD) by virus isolation is complicated by the fact that very few strains of IBD virus grow in cell cultures and not all strains grow in eggs. The only reliable method of IBD virus isolation is by inoculation of specific pathogen free chickens, which is obviously inconvenient and time consuming. Direct immunofluorescent staining of bursal impression smears provide an easy,

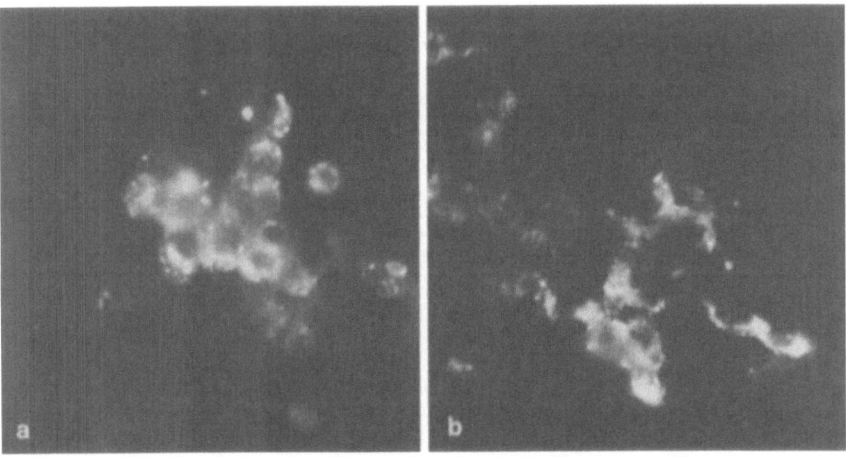

Fig. 3   Respiratory syncytial virus antigens in (a) impression smear
and (b) cryostat section of pneumonic calf lung.

rapid and sensitive means of detecting the virus (Allan et al., 1984b).
Newcastle disease virus and infectious laryngo-tracheitis virus are not difficult to isolate in either cell cultures or eggs. However these viruses
cause diseases which are notifiable in Northern Ireland. Rapid diagnosis
is important because it enables control measures to be put into effect as
soon as possible. This is critical in controlling the spread of Newcastle
disease, in which large amounts of virus become airborne and can be carried
for miles on the wind. Although less sensitive than virus isolation, immunofluorescent staining of cryostat sections of trachea can be used for
rapid diagnosis of both these diseases. Fluorescence occurs in the tracheal
epithelial cells.

Recognition of the growth of 'difficult'/non-cytopathogenic viruses in various culture systems

Immunofluorescent staining of allantoic cells has been used in this
laboratory for over a decade for isolating and detecting growth of avian
infectious bronchitis (IB) virus in eggs (Fig. 4). Immunofluorescence has
several advantages over the standard embryo dwarfing test as a criterion
for the detection of IB virus. It is a specific test whereas dwarfing is
not. It can be carried out in half the time required for dwarfing and few-
er eggs are required. Furthermore, immunofluorescence is more sensitive
because many isolates of IB virus require 4 to 8 embryo passages before they
produce dwarfing. In contrast, only 2 embryo passages are generally

required for diagnosis by immunofluorescence (Clarke et al., 1972).

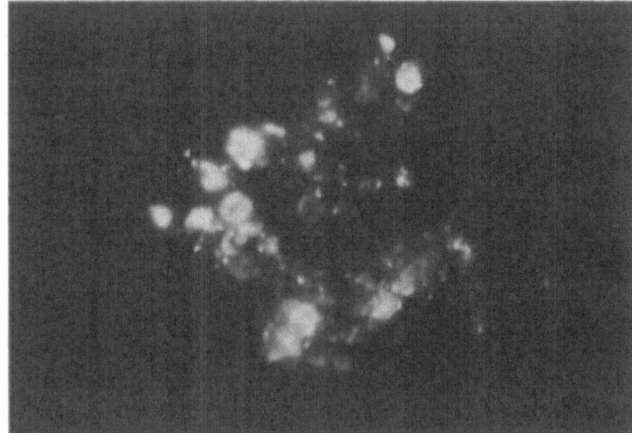

Fig. 4   Avian infectious bronchitis antigens in allantoic cells of eggs inoculated with tracheal material from pullets with respiratory disease.

While some bovine respiratory viruses eg RSV and coronavirus are difficult to isolate in cell cultures, isolation attempts in bovine tracheal organ cultures are often successful.   Neither RSV nor coronavirus causes ciliastasis.   However growth of these viruses in tracheal organ cultures can be monitored by immunofluorescent staining of cells harvested from the culture media (Fig. 5).

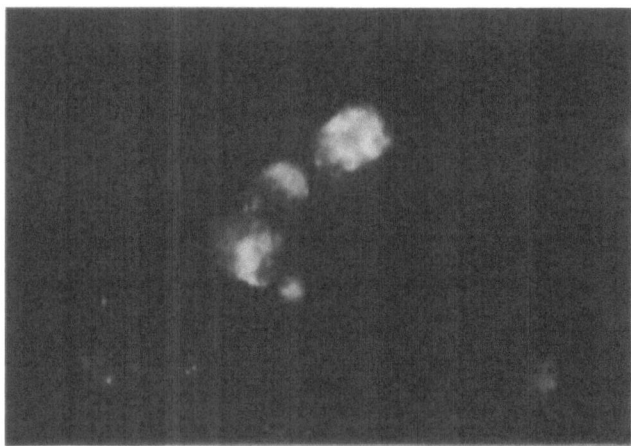

Fig. 5   Coronavirus antigens in cells harvested from bovine tracheal organ culture inoculated with lung material from calves with respiratory disease.

BVD virus is one of the commonest bovine viruses isolated in this laboratory. This virus is also a frequent contaminant of foetal bovine serum and hence also of many cell cultures. As mentioned above, most isolates of BVD virus are non-cytopathogenic. Immunofluorescent staining of susceptible cell cultures inoculated with suspect material is the best way of detecting these viruses. Immunofluorescence due to BVD virus is characteristically diffuse and often dull (Fig. 6). The choice of objective

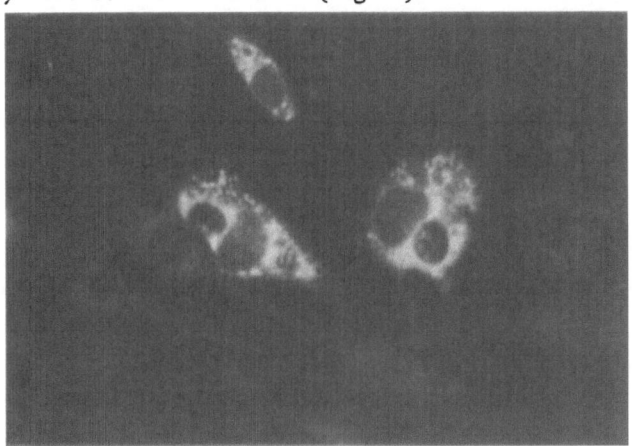

Fig. 6   BVD virus antigens in foetal bovine lung cells.

lens is critical here. BVD virus immunofluorescence detected with a X40 lens with a numerical aperture of 1.30 is not always visible using a X40 lens with a numerical aperture of 0.65.

Rotaviruses have proved difficult to adapt to growth in cell cultures using conventional techniques. However, by treating faecal specimens containing rotavirus with trypsin, some, but not all rotaviruses can be grown serially in cell cultures. Immunofluorescence has proved invaluable in monitoring the growth of these isolates (Fig. 7), most of which are non-cytopathogenic. Immunofluorescence has also been used to recognise isolates of atypical rotavirus ie those which lack the conventional rotavirus group antigen (McNulty et al., 1981).

Detection of viral antibodies by indirect immunofluorescence

Viral antibodies can be rapidly and fairly simply demonstrated by indirect immunofluorescence. The viral antigen is reacted with the serum under test and counterstained with the appropriate FITC-conjugated antispecies immunoglobulin. In general, this test detects antibodies directed against both type and group antigens of a particular virus. The broad

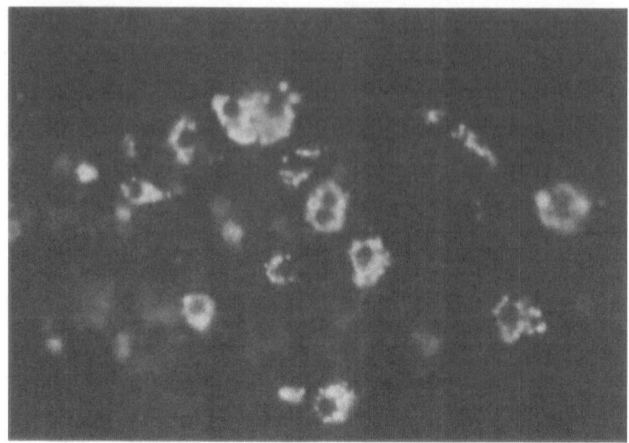

Fig. 7   Rotavirus antigens in chick embryo liver cells inoculated
with faecal material from 3 week old broiler chickens.

specificity afforded by reaction with group antigens makes indirect immunofluorescence very useful for survey purposes. Furthermore, indirect immunofluorescence is sensitive eg a microtitre indirect immunofluorescence test
detected antibodies to adenovirus in 70.8% of 595 avain field sera, whereas
the standard agar gel immunodiffusion test detected antibodies in only
52.6% of these sera (Adair et al., 1980). Similarly, indirect immunofluorescence has been shown to be more sensitive than the serum neutralisation test for detecting antibodies to infectious laryngo-tracheitis virus
and the haemagglutination inhibition tests for bovine parainfluenza virus
type 3 and Egg Drop Syndrome adenovirus (B M Adair, personal communication).

Indirect immunofluorescence provides a convenient method for detecting
antibodies to non-cytopathogenic viruses eg rotaviruses (McNulty et al.,
1979, 1984a). Cryostat sections of infected tissues can also be used as a
source of viral antigens, so the method can also be used for viruses which
have not been adapted to growth in cell cultures.

Another application of indirect immunofluorescence is to look for
evidence of infection in animal species from which a particular virus has
not yet been isolated. Thus, although neither coronaviruses nor pneumo-
viruses have been isolated from sheep, we have found antibody reacting with
bovine enteric coronavirus and bovine RSV in sheep sera. The staining pattern obtained with sera from 'heterologous' animal species may differ from
that seen with sera from the 'homologous' species. For example, most ovine
sera do not react with the 'flecks' of viral antigen on and outside the

plasma membranes of cells infected with bovine RSV, but stain only the cytoplasmic inclusions. This suggests that the pneumovirus which infects sheep
shares a nucleocapsid antigen with bovine RSV, but has different surface
antigens.

Recognition of new viruses

The way in which immunofluorescence has been used in the recognition
of previously unknown virus infections is illustrated below.

During investigation of outbreaks of infectious runting in broiler
chickens, small round viruses resembling enteroviruses were detected by
electron microscopy in the faeces of birds from affected flocks during the
first week of life. However attempts to isolate these viruses in cell cultures were unsuccessful. This suggested that these viruses might be bacter-
iophages rather than animal viruses. In an attempt to answer this question,
the small round viruses were partially purified from infected faeces and an
antiserum to them was prepared in chickens and conjugated with FITC. This
conjugate was then used to look for small round virus antigens in chickens
orally inoculated with faecal suspensions containing the virus. Specific
immunofluorescence was observed in the villous epithelial cells of the
small intestine (Fig. 8). The specificity of this immunofluorescence was

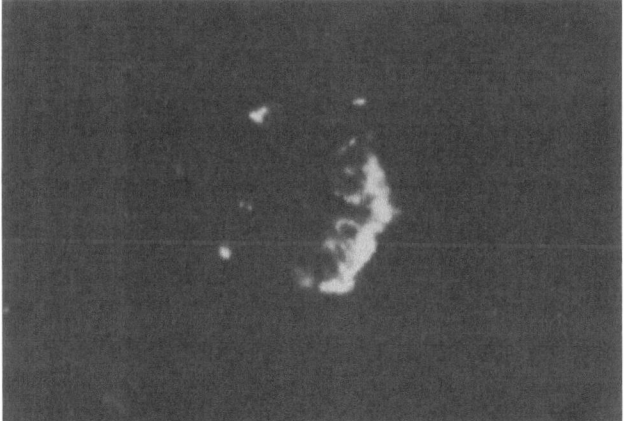

Fig. 8   Immunofluorescence in villous epithelial cells of jejunum of
broiler chicken orally inoculated with an enterovirus-like agent associated with the runting syndrome.

confirmed by thin section electron microscopy, which revealed crystalline
aggregates of enterovirus-like particles in the cytoplasm of enterocytes.
Further characterisation of the small round virus indicates that it appears

to be a previously unknown chicken enterovirus (McNulty et al., 1984b).

The detection in sheep of antibodies reacting with bovine enteric coronavirus antigens has been described above. A FITC-conjugated antiserum to bovine enteric coronavirus has been used to look for coronavirus antigens in necropsy material from sheep. So far, only a small number of ovine carcases has been available for examination. However, immunofluorescence has been detected in the cytoplasm of bronchiolar epithelial cells of a lamb with pneumonia. This provides further evidence for coronavirus infection in sheep.

REFERENCES

Adair, B.M., McFerran, J.B. and Calvert, V.M. 1980. Development of a micro-titre fluorescent antibody test for serological detection of adeno-virus infection in birds. Avian Pathol., 9, 291-300.

Allan, G.M., McNulty, M.S., McCracken, R.M. and McFerran, J.B. 1984a. Rapid diagnosis of Aujeszky's disease in pigs by immunofluorescence. Res. Vet. Sci., in press.

Allan, G.M., McNulty, M.S., Connor, T.J., McCracken, R.M. and McFerran, J.B. 1984b. Rapid diagnosis of infectious bursal disease infection by immunofluorescence on clinical material. Avian Pathol., in press.

Clarke, J.K., McFerran, J.B. and Gay, F.W. 1972. Use of allantoic cells for the detection of avian infectious bronchitis virus. Archiv. ges. Virusforsch., 36, 62-70.

Gardner, P.S. and McQuillin, J. 1980. Rapid Virus Diagnosis: Application of Immunofluorescence. 2nd edition. (Butterworths, London).

McNulty, M.S., Allan, G.M., Todd, D. and McFerran, J.B. 1979. Isolation and cell culture propagation of rotaviruses from turkeys and chickens. Arch. Virol., 61, 13-21.

McNulty, M.S., Allan, G.M., Todd, D., McFerran, J.B. and McCracken, R.M. 1981. Isolation from chickens of a rotavirus lacking the rotavirus group antigen. J. gen. Virol., 55, 405-413.

McNulty, M.S., Bryson, D.G. and Allan, G.M. 1983. Experimental respiratory syncytial virus pneumonia in young calves: Microbiologic and immuno-fluorescence findings. Am. J. Vet. Res., 44, 1656-1659.

McNulty, M.S., Allan, G.M. and McFerran, J.B. 1984a. Prevalence of anti-body to conventional and atypical rotaviruses in chickens. Vet. Rec., in press.

McNulty, M.S., Allan, G.M., Connor, T.J., McFerran, J.B. and McCracken, R.M. 1984b. An entero-like virus associated with the runting syndrome in broiler chickens. Avian Pathol., in press.

TAGGING OF VIRAL ANTIGENS USING IMMUNOPEROXIDASE AND IMMUNOGOLD TECHNIQUES

R. Ducatelle[o], F. Castryck[oo], J. Hoorens[o]
[o]Department of Veterinary Pathology, State University of Gent, Belgium
[oo]Veterinary Investigation Centre Torhout, Belgium

ABSTRACT

An unlabelled immunoperoxidase method on paraffin sections was used for the diagnosis of pseudorabies (Aujeszky's disease) in 78 young pigs. The sensitivity and specificity of this new diagnostic method was compared to that of conventional diagnostic methods, namely virus isolation, immuno-fluorescence and histopathology. It was found that this immunoperoxidase method was specific and sensitive and therefore can be used as an alter-native diagnostic method. A limited number of cases also were tested with an indirect immunogold method on paraffin sections. This method was specific but inferior in sensitivity as compared to the immunoperoxidase method. The possibilities, advantages and disadvantages of both immuno-peroxidase and immunogold methods are discussed.

INTRODUCTION

Immunolabelling of viral antigens in tissue sections is usually done with fluorescein-conjugated antibodies.

In order to obviate some of the deficiencies and limitations of immuno-fluorescence techniques, new marker techniques to make antigen - antibody reactions visible have been developed in the last 15 years. These techniques are enzyme-conjugated antibody methods. The enzyme most widely used for this purpose is the plant enzyme horseradish peroxidase. Immuno-peroxidase methods are generally used in combination with the diamino-benzidine hydrogen peroxide method of Graham and Karnovsky (1966). A direct and an indirect immunoperoxidase method (IpX) can be used. Both methods are analogous to the direct and the indirect immunofluorescence methods. At present direct and indirect IpX are used extensively in the veterinary field for early detection of virus multiplication in cell cultures (Bartoszcze and Roszkowski, 1979; Krishnaswamy et al., 1981; Chasey, 1981; Sutmoller and Cowan, 1974). Aujeszky's disease virus multiplication eg can be detected as early as 8 h post inoculation (Bartoszcze, 1982).

Since 1970, an unlabelled three step IpX method called peroxidase-antiperoxidase method (PAP), has been developed (Sternberger et al., 1970). It offers the advantage of being easily applicable to paraffin sections of fixed animal tissues (Sternberger, 1974). This highly sensitive method has until recently been used almost exclusively for the qualitative study of hormones in brain tissue and of immunoglobulins in various tissues of man and animals (review: Ducatelle and Hoorens, 1980). The demonstration of viral antigens in paraffin sections of fixed tissues with this PAP method has gained significant interest only in the last three years (Ducatelle et al., 1980; Carthew and Sparrow, 1981; Chu et al., 1982; Ducatelle et al., 1982; Miry et al., 1983), although this possibility already had been investigated ten years ago (Di Stefano et al., 1973).

The present report is a first account of the value of the unlabelled IpX method for diagnostic purposes by comparison with immunofluorescence on cryostat sections and virus isolation in cell cultures. These tests were made on diagnostic material from pigs with suspected Aujeszky's disease.

Preliminary tests also were performed to evaluate colloidal gold as a marker for viral antigens at the light microscopic level.

MATERIALS AND METHODS

1. Materials

Seventy-eight pigs, ranging in age from fetal to 10 weeks old, were included in this study. These were all autopsy cases which were clinically suspected of Aujeszky's disease. The animals were usually autopsied within the first 24 h post-mortem. At autopsy, as a rule two adjacent specimens were sampled from each of the following tissues: transverse slices of the cerebral cortex near the sulcus centralis, transverse slices of cerebellum through the vermis, and longitudinal slices through the brain stem. Samples were also taken from the tonsils and from the lungs. Each time, one of two specimens was frozen for cryostat sectioning, while the other specimen was fixed in 10% phosphate buffered formalin for paraffin embedding. After at least 24 h formalin fixation, the tissues were dehydrated through a graded series of alcohol, cleared in xylene and embedded in paraffin (Tissue wax TSW20, Medite, West Germany; melting point 56° to $58^{\circ}C$).

The rest of the brain and the tonsils were taken for virus isolation.

2. Methods

The original unlabelled immunoperoxidase staining method for the demonstration of pseudorabies viral antigens in paraffin sections (Ducatelle et al., 1982) has been further developed in order to improve the repro-ducibility of the method for routine diagnosis.

2.1. Immune sera:

New Zealand White rabbits were used for the production of hyperimmune serum against Aujeszky's disease virus. The animals were injected 4 times subcutaneously using 5 pig doses of commercial inactivated virus vaccine (Geskyvac, Laboratoire Roger Bellon) and 4 times using 5 pig doses of commercial live vaccine (Duvaxyn Aujeszky, Duphar), each time with 3 week intervals. Three weeks after the last injection, the animals were challenged subcutaneously with 0.5 ml 10^6 $TCID_{50}$/ml live virulent Aujeszky's disease virus strain 75V19 (Pensaert et al., 1980). The survivors were further immunised with commercial live vaccine with 3 week intervals, until a mean serum neutralising antibody titre of 512 was obtained. Antibody titres were determined at the virology laboratory as described by Pensaert et al. (1980). Blood samples from these rabbits were collected 10 days after the last booster vaccination. The globulin fraction of the pooled sera was isolated by ammonium sulphate precipitation and dialysis against phosphate buffer at pH 6.3.

Antiserum to rabbit globulins was raised in goats. The animals were injected with 0.3 g of rabbit globulins and 0.5 ml of complete Freund's adjuvant every 3 weeks for a period of 4 months. Thereafter they were boosted every 6 weeks. Blood samples were taken one week after vaccination.

Anti-peroxidase serum was raised in New Zealand White rabbits. The rabbits were injected with 10,000 units of horseradish peroxidase (Type 2, Sigma, St. Louis, USA) and 0.5 ml complete Freund's adjuvant every 4 weeks for a period of 6 months. They were bled 10 days after the last injection. Using this anti-peroxidase, a soluble complex was made with horseradish peroxidase according to the method of Sternberger, modified by Vandesande (1978).

2.2. Immunoperoxidase staining procedure:

5μm paraffin sections from all tissue blocks were cut and stained with an unlabelled antibody-enzyme method (Ducatelle et al., 1980). For this purpose the sections were first deparaffinated and rehydrated. All incubations with sera were done in a moist chamber at 25°C. Between each incubation the sections were washed for 5 mins in a 0.01 M tris buffered saline solution at pH 7.6 on a shaker platform.

The sections were first incubated with undiluted normal goat serum for 20 mins. Thereafter the primary rabbit antiserum to Aujeszky's disease virus was used 1/800 diluted with 0.01 M tris buffered saline at pH 8.2.

This incubation was done for 2 h. Goat - anti rabbit globulin serum, diluted 1/30 with tris buffer at pH 7.6, was put on the sections for 20 mins. Finally, the peroxidase - antiperoxidase complex was used for 20 mins. It was diluted 1/300 in tris buffer at pH 7.6. After incubation with the sera, the sections were immersed for 5 to 7 mins in a jar containing the staining solution. This solution consisted of 0.005% H_2O_2 and 0.01% 3,3 '-diamino-benzidine-HCl in 0.05 M tris-HCl buffer at pH 7.6.

After staining the sections were dehydrated and mounted with clear-mount.

In each batch of 20 immunoperoxidase stained sections, a control positive and negative section from an experimentally infected piglet and a control non-infected piglet respectively were included. Control of the procedure was done on sections of positive material, taking the sections through the incubation series, but each time omitting one of the sera. Control of endogenous peroxidase activity was done by bringing sections in the staining solution without prior incubation with sera.

2.3. Immunofluorescence staining:

8 μm cryostat sections from all frozen specimens were stained with a direct immunofluorescence technique using fluorescein labelled antiserum to Aujeszky's disease virus prepared in swine at a dilution of 1/5 to 1/30.

2.4. Virus isolation:

Virus isolation from all pigs was done by inoculating tissue homogenates onto primary pig kidney cells at the virology laboratory of Prof. M.B. Pensaert and at the National Institute of Veterinary Research as described (Pensaert et al., 1980).

2.5. Histologic staining:

Paraffin sections cut adjacent to the immunoperoxidase stained paraffin sections were deparaffinated and stained with haematoxylin and eosin (HE) and luxol fast blue - periodic acid schiff when appropriate (Luna, 1968).

2.6. Immunogold staining:

Paraffin sections adjacent to the immunoperoxidase and histologic stained sections from 5 positive and 2 negative cases were used for immunogold staining. The sections were prepared as for immunoperoxidase staining. Pre-incubation with undiluted normal goat serum and incubation with primary anti-Aujeszky serum also were similar to the immunoperoxidase technique. However, the optimal dilution of anti-Aujeszky serum here was 1/400.

Thereafter the sections were rinsed in 0.01 M tris buffered saline at pH 7.6 and subsequently incubated for 2 h with goat antibodies to rabbit immunoglobulin linked to 20 nm colloidal gold particles (GAR G20, Janssen, Beerse, Belgium). This antiserum was diluted 1/10 in 0.1% bovine serum albumen and centrifuged for 10 mins at 250 xg immediately before use. There-after, the sections were rinsed, dehydrated and mounted as for immuno-peroxidase staining.

RESULTS

The immunoperoxidase technique yielded reliable and constantly re-producible results. The application of the immunoperoxidase technique did not cause significant technical difficulties, so that it could be learned by any laboratory technician in a relatively short time.

After immunoperoxidase staining of paraffin sections, cells infected with Aujeszky's disease virus contained a brown fine granular staining product. This staining product was strictly confined to the cells. Both the nucleus and the cytoplasm or the cytoplasm alone or the nucleus alone could be seen stained brown. The interstitium showed a very faint overall background staining, giving a yellowish tinge to the sections. The distri-bution of stain throughout various tissues was similar to that described earlier in a study on the relation between histopathology and immuno-peroxidase staining of paraffin sections (Ducatelle et al., 1982).

In non-infected tissues the brown staining was not present. Neverthe-less, these tissues did contain a yellowish-brown colour where red blood cells were present. Endogenous peroxidase activity of leucocytes was not seen. Background staining was similar to sections of infected tissues.

The results of the double-blind comparative study of immunofluorescence, virus isolation, histologic staining and immunoperoxidase staining are represented in Table 1. There was complete agreement between the results yielded by the 4 methods in 63 out of the 78 cases studied. In 8 cases, a positive result given by one method was not substantiated using the other 3 methods.

The criteria used for the interpretation of histologic staining (HE) were those outlined earlier (Ducatelle et al., 1982). These criteria essentially required the presence of foci of necrosis and presence of either eosinophylic or amphophylic intranuclear inclusion bodies in association with these foci. In sections of the central nervous system, non-suppurative encephalitic lesions should be present.

TABLE 1   Comparative diagnostic study of porcine pseudorabies.

IF	VI	HE	PAP	N°
-	-	-	-	34
+	+	+	+	29
+	+	+	-	2
+	+	-	+	2
+	-	+	+	2
-	+	+	+	0
+	+	-	-	0
+	-	-	+	1
+	-	+	-	0
+	-	-	-	2
-	+	-	-	2
-	-	+	-	2
-	-	-	+	2
				78

VI = Virus isolation.
IF = Immunofluorescence.
HE = Histologic examination.
PAP = Immunoperoxidase.

After immunogold staining of paraffin sections, a number of cells were clearly stained pink. The sections showed no background staining. Red blood cells were refringent but not stained brown. White blood cells were not visible. When comparing these sections with adjacent serial immuno-peroxidase-stained sections, it was obvious though that not all positive cells were stained with colloidal gold, or at least that the gold tone was not sufficient to be perceptible under the light microscope.

DISCUSSION
From Table 1 can be concluded that virus isolation, immunofluorescent staining of cryostat sections, immunoperoxidase staining of paraffin

sections and histologic staining of paraffin sections can all yield reliable diagnostic results when properly used for the diagnosis of Aujeszky's disease in piglets. Immunoperoxidase staining of paraffin sections can thus be considered a useful alternative diagnostic method for this purpose.

This technique nevertheless has some serious disadvantages. It is much more time consuming than immunofluorescence, since it first requires a paraffin embedding and thereafter a long series of incubations with sera. These incubations with several sera demand many manipulations, thus holding a significant risk of technical errors and non-specific reactions (Bergroth et al., 1980; Fan, 1980). Finally, immunoperoxidase staining of paraffin sections suffers from the same disadvantage as any other technique on tissue sections, namely that one only examines a very small portion of tissue in only one plane. This inconvenience can be overcome in part by cutting semi-serial sections and by taking several tissue specimens.

Immunoperoxidase staining of paraffin sections also offers a number of important advantages (Vandesande, 1979). The most important advantage is that it can be applied to fixed tissue specimens. This is particularly of interest when diagnostic material has to be transported a long way under adverse conditions of climate. The Sternberger immunoperoxidase technique also opens up new possibilities for retrospective studies on stored fixed tissues. This is being done at present with cases of Aujeszky's disease encephalitis (Reinacher and Fraze, pers. commun.).

As to the technical aspects of this method, the application of the immunoperoxidase technique to the tissue sections yielded reproducible results and therefore did not require pretreatment of the tissue sections with pepsin or trypsin (Dell'Orto et al., 1982). Sera were usually stored at -70°C. Sera in use could be kept for 1 to 2 weeks when stored at 4°C. This period could be significantly prolonged when adding 0.02 g of sodium azide per 100 ml of serum (Sofroniew and Schrell, 1982). Since endogenous peroxidase activity was very low, it was unnecessary to block this enzyme (Straus, 1972).

The Sternberger peroxidase - antiperoxidase immunohistochemical staining method has been claimed to be highly sensitive not only for the demonstration of hormones in paraffin sections of central nervous tissue (Moriarty et al., 1973), but also for the demonstration of immunoglobulins in a variety of tissues, eg also in pig tissues (Brown et al., 1974). The technique is said to be highly insensitive to long-term fixation of the tissues (Celio, 1979) and to paraffin embedding (Halmi, 1978). In the present material, which was used for the demonstration of virus antigens, the optimal dilution of the anti-Aujeszky's virus serum was 1/800 but positive staining was still perceptible at a 1/6000 dilution. This is far beyond dilutions used for other immunologic techniques on tissue sections.

The immunogold technique is a newcomer in the group of immunohisto-chemical methods which are applicable to tissue sections. It was first developed for the demonstration of antigens under the electron microscope (Horisberger and Vonlanthen, 1977), where it can even be used for the simultaneous demonstration of multiple antigens (Larsson, 1979). It has only recently been described as a method for the light microscopic staining of antigens in paraffin sections (Gu et al., 1981). Pseudorabies virus can be demonstrated in ultra-thin sections of infected cell cultures using col-loidal gold-labelled staphylococcal protein A (Weiland, 1981). In the present study, Aujeszky's disease virus was demonstrated in paraffin sections of pig tissues using colloidal gold labelled antibodies. Nevertheless, the labelling was obviously incomplete, leaving a lot of antigens unlabelled, or insufficiently labelled to be visible with the naked eye. Consequently, this indirect immunogold technique is at present not yet useful as a diag-nostic method for pseudorabies in swine in our hands. Further developments of the technique will probably make it a useful diagnostic method, because of several advantages. The method is shorter and thus less time consuming and less subject to technical errors. The method is also directly trans-ferable to the ultrastructural level, consequently allowing investigation of structures and lesions in more detail. Finally, this method is not influ-enced by endogenous peroxidase or pseudoperoxidase activity in the tissues. The application of silver-toning on colloidal gold stained sections may markedly enhance the contrast and thus improve the sensitivity of immunogold staining for light microscopy (Done, pers. commun.). Future applications of colloidal gold labelling methods on tissue sections will probably lie in the examination of dual or multiple virus infections and in the study of early stages of virus morphogenesis.

ACKNOWLEDGEMENTS

The authors thank Prof. M.B. Pensaert and Dr. R. Biront for virus isolations. Mr. P. Degroot and Miss M. Carpentier, Mrs L. van Overschelde and Mr. D. Dugardeyn are acknowledged for their technical assistance.

REFERENCES

Bartoszcze, M. and Roszkowski, J. 1979. The use of the indirect immuno-
peroxidase method for the detection of Aujeszky's disease virus in
cell culture. Zbl. Vet. Med. B., 26, 253-256.
Bartoszcze, M. 1981. Immunoenzyme techniques for diagnosis of Aujeszky's
virus infections. Zeszyty Naukowe Akademii Rolniczo-Technicznei w
Olsztynie, Weterynaria, 13, 53-87.
Bergroth, V., Reitamo, S., Konttinen, Y.T. and Lalla, M. 1980. Sensitivity
and nonspecific staining of various immunoperoxidase techniques.
Histochem., 68, 17-22.
Brown, P., Bourne, J. and Steel, M. 1974. Immunoperoxidase and immuno-
fluorescence techniques in pig tissues. Histochem., 40, 343-348.
Carthew, P. and Sparrow, S. 1981. Murine coronaviruses: the histopathology
of disease induced by intranasal inoculation. Res. Vet. Sci., 30,
270-273.
Celio, M.R. 1979. Immunohistochemistry on Bouin-fixed fetal tissue, stored
for thirty years in ethanol. Histochem., 61, 347-350.
Chasey, D. 1980. A simple and rapid immunoperoxidase test for the detection of virus antigens in tissue culture. Vet. Rec., 106, 506-507.
Chu, R.M., Li, N.J., Glock, R.D. and Ross, R.F. 1982. Applications of
peroxidase-antiperoxidase staining technique for detection of transmissible gastroenteritis virus in pigs. Am. J. Vet. Res., 43, 77-81.
Dell'Orto, P., Viale, G., Colombi, R., Braidotti, P. and Coggi, G. 1982.
Immunohistochemical localisation of human immunoglobulins and Lysozyme
in epoxy-embedded lymph nodes. J. Histochem. Cytochem., 30, 630-636.
Di Stefano, H.S., Marucci, A.A. and Dougherty, R.M. 1973. Immunohisto-
chemical demonstration of avian leukosis virus antigens in paraffin
embedded tissue. Proc. Soc. Exp. Biol. Med., 142, 1111-1113.
Ducatelle, R., Coussement, W. and Hoorens, J. 1980. Demonstration of
canine distemper viral antigen in paraffin sections, using an unlabelled antibody-enzyme method. Am. J. Vet. Res., 41, 1860-1862.
Ducatelle, R. and Hoorens, J. 1980. Immunoperoxidase staining techniques
and their application in veterinary science. Vlaams Diergen.
Tijdschr., 49, 100-113.
Ducatelle, R., Coussement, W. and Hoorens, J. 1982. Immunoperoxidase
study of Aujeszky's disease in pigs. Res. Vet. Sci., 32, 294-302.
Fan, K. 1980. High affinity binding of horseradish peroxidase to collagen-
ous tissue in formalin-paraffin processed human tissue. Stain Tech.,
55, 307-311.
Graham, R.C. and Karnovsky, M.J. 1966. The early stages of absorption of
injected horseradish peroxidase in the proximal tubules of mouse
kidney: ultrastructural cytochemistry by a new technique. J. Histochem. Cytochem., 14, 291-302.
Gu, J., De Mey, J., Moeremans, M. and Polak, J.M. 1981. Sequential use of
the PAP and immunogold staining methods for the light microscopical
double staining of tissue antigens. Regulatory Peptides,1, 365-374.
Halmi, N.S. 1978. Immunostaining of growth hormone and prolactin in
paraffin-embedded and stored or previously stained materials. J.
Histochem. Cytochem., 26, 486-495.
Horisberger, M. and Vonlanthen, M. 1977. Location of mannan and chitin on
thin sections of budding yeasts with gold markers. Arch. Microbiol.,
115, 1-7.
Krishnaswamy, S., Keshavamurthy, B.S. and Sundararajan, S. 1981. The use
of the direct immunoperoxidase test to detect the multiplication of
rinderpest virus in bovine kidney cell culture. Vet. Microbiol., 6,
23-29.

36

Larsson, L.I. 1979. Simultaneous ultrastructural demonstration of multiple peptides in endocrine cells by a novel immunocytochemical method. Nature, 282, 743-746.

Luna, L.G. 1968. Manual of histologic staining methods of the armed forces institute of pathology. 3rd. Edition. (McGraw-Hill Book Company, New York).

Miry, C., Ducatelle, R., Thoonen, H. and Hoorens, J. 1983. Immunoperoxidase study of canine distemper virus pneumonia. Res. Vet. Sci., 34, 145-148.

Moriarty, G.C., Moriarty, C.M. and Sternberger, L.A. 1973. Ultrastructural immunocytochemistry with unlabelled antibodies and the peroxidase-antiperoxidase complex. A technique more sensitive than radioimmuno-assay. J. Histochem. Cytochem., 21, 825-833.

Pensaert, M.B., Commeyne, S. and Andries, K. 1980. Vaccination of dogs against pseudorabies (Aujeszky's disease), using an inactivated-virus vaccine. Am. J. Vet. Res., 41, 2016-2019.

Sofroniew, M.V. and Schrell, U. 1982. Long-term storage and regular repeated use of diluted antisera in glass staining jars for increased sensitivity, reproducibility, and convenience of single- and two-color light microscopic immunocytochemistry. J. Histochem. Cytochem. 30, 504-511.

Sternberger, L.A., Hardy, P.H., Cuculis, J.J. and Meyer, H.G. 1970. The unlabelled antibody enzyme method of immunohistochemistry. Preparation and properties of soluble antigen-antibody complex and its use in identification of spirochetes. J. Histochem. Cytochem., 18, 315-333.

Sternberger, L.A. 1974. Immunocytochemistry. (John Wiley and Sons, New York).

Straus, W. 1972. Phenylhydrazine; use in immunoperoxidase procedures. J. Histochem. Cytochem., 20, 949-951.

Sutmoller, P. and Cowan, K.M. 1974. The detection of foot- and mouth disease virus antigens in infected cell cultures by immunoperoxidase techniques. J. Gen. Virol., 22, 287-291.

Vandesande, F. 1978. Immunohistochemisch onderzoek van het hypothalamo-hypofysair systeem bij het rund, de rat, de brattleboro rat en de kikker, met anti-oxytocine, anti-mesotocine, anti-vasotocine, anti-vasopressine, anti-runderneurofysine I en anti-runderneurofysine II antiserum. Proefschrift.

Vandesande, F. 1979. A critical review of immunocytochemical methods for light microscopy. J. Neurosci. Methods, 1, 3-23.

Weiland, F. 1981. Ultrastructural visualisation of virus-antibody binding by means of colloidal gold-protein A. Ann. Virol. (Inst. Pasteur), 132, 549-556.

DETECTION OF BVD VIRUS IN VIREMIC CATTLE
BY AN INDIRECT IMMUNOPEROXIDASE TECHNIQUE

A. Meyling

State Veterinary Serum Laboratory
Bulowsvej 27
DK 1870 Copenhagen V
Denmark

ABSTRACT

An indirect peroxidase staining technique (PO) for detection of BVD-virus in the serum of infected cattle has been developed. The test, which is performed in microtitre plates is at least as sensitive as the fluorescent antibody technique (FA) and is easier to perform and read. The reagents in the PO test are a hyperimmune anti-BVD-virus serum raised in a goat by immunising with BVD virus grown in goat cells. Peroxidase-labelled immuno-purified bovine antibodies to goat IgG are used in the second step. BVD virus was demonstrated in 12 (0.9%) of 1332 normally randomly collected cattle sera from 2 slaughterhouses, 1042 (78%) of these had neutralising antibodies to BVD virus. Of 363 cattle from 13 herds that had recently experienced losses due to BVD, 317 (87%) had antibodies to BVD, but of the 46 seronegative animals 38 (83%) were found to be viremic. In animals with clinical disease, titres of BVD virus as assayed by PO staining were found to be as high as $10^{5.5}$ $TCID_{50}$/0.01 ml serum. The mean titre of animals with disease was found to be $10^{3.1}$ $TCID_{50}$/0.01 ml and $10^{2.6}$ $TCID_{50}$/0.01 ml for apparently healthy animals. The PO staining technique for detection of BVD virus is a practical test for detection of viremic animals in infected herds and for diagnosing cases of BVD.

INTRODUCTION

Bovine viral diarrhoea (BVD) virus is a very commonly occurring pathogen in cattle. It belongs to the genus pestivirus and is antigenically closely related to the viruses of hog cholera (HC) and border disease (BD). Some strains of BVD virus are cytopathogenic (CP) but many, like other members of the genus pestivirus, are non-cytopathogenic (NCP).

In the past, several methods have been developed for the detection and titration of NCP BVD virus. These methods are based on interference between NCP and CP strains of BVD virus or inhibition of an antiviral compound (Gillespie et al., 1962; Maisonnave and Rossi, 1982).

The fluorescent antibody (FA) technique has been used for many years for detection and identification of BVD virus. However, often the diffuse cytoplasmic fluorescence of NCP BVD virus is quite weak and it is therefore difficult if not impossible to adapt the FA technique for BVD virus to the microtitre system.

Recently an enzyme-conjugated antibody assay for detection of antibodies to BVD and HC viruses in swine serum has been described (Saunders, 1977; Jensen, 1981), and an indirect peroxidase (PO) technique has been developed for detection of BVD virus in tissues of infected animals (Ohmann, 1983).

The present report describes the use of indirect PO staining for detection of BVD virus in cell cultures and the technique is especially designed to detect BVD virus in the serum of infected animals.

The use of serum for inoculation of tissue cultures in connection with diagnosis of viremia in BVD is relevant, since this condition, so far as the fatal cases are concerned, is associated with immunologic unresponsiveness and absence of neutralising antibodies to the BVD virus causing the disease (Steck et al., 1981). The same applies to the apparently healthy animals with persistent viremia (Coria and McClurkin, 1978). In experimentally infected animals, viremia occurs for several days before and until neutralising antibodies become detectable. Isolation of BVD virus from serum and leucocytes from such animals is also described in this report.

MATERIALS AND METHODS

Blood samples

1332 blood samples collected randomly at 2 slaughterhouses and submitted to the laboratory under the bovine leucosis eradication scheme, 363 blood samples from 13 herds that had experienced losses due to BVD, and 1313 diagnostic blood samples from cattle suspected of being affected with BVD and submitted to the laboratory by practising veterinarians, were examined for neutralising antibodies to BVD virus and for BVD virus by the microtitre PO staining technique described below.

The titre of BVD virus in 70 diagnostic blood samples from clinically affected animals and in 70 samples from apparently healthy animals in herds that had experienced losses due to BVD was determined after the samples had been stored from 1 to 12 months at -20°C. Tenfold dilutions of serum in Eagle's minimal essential medium (MEM) containing 5% calf serum were made and 10 μl of the dilution were added to each of two wells in microtitre trays. BVD virus was demonstrated by PO staining as described below and titres calculated according to Karber. In addition to these sera, bimonthly drawn samples from two persistently infected animals were treated likewise.

Ninety-six samples and the same number of EDTA-stabilised whole blood samples drawn daily from 8 calves that had been experimentally exposed to 2 field strains of BVD virus were examined virologically. These experimentally infected calves had been used as unvaccinated controls in a vaccine trial.

Buffy coat cells were prepared from each sample by centrifugation (1000 x g) for 20 min. Plasma was removed and the leucocyte rich layer recovered. The cells were washed three times in PBS and resuspended in Eagle's MEM in a volume corresponding to 50% of the sample. Cell suspensions were frozen twice and in parallel with corresponding serum samples used to inoculate calf testis (CT) cultures, which were subsequently processed for FA staining.

Tissue cultures

A bovine kidney cell line, BK347 (kindly supplied by Fort Dodge Laboratories) was used for virus isolation and subsequent PO staining and also for serum neutralisation tests. CT cells used for seeding 24 well plates for FA staining of BVD virus were prepared from calves belonging to the institute herd, which is free of BVD virus infection. BK347 cells and CT cells were grown in Eagle's MEM supplemented with 10% calf serum. The serum used for tissue culture medium was prepared from the blood of one calf reared and kept in a unit isolated from the other animals of the institute herd.

Immune sera and conjugates

Hyperimmune sera to a Danish cytopathogenic strain of BVD virus (VD 133) were raised in a 3-month-old calf and a 1-year-old goat from the institute herd. Testis cultures derived from the animals' own organs and grown in medium supplemented with homologous serum free of both BVD virus and antibody were inoculated with virus. Infected cells were recovered in an amount of PBS equal to 1/100 of the original volume. After 2 freeze-thaw cycles and sonication for 10 sec. on ice the cell debris was removed by centrifugation (5000 x g). The supernatants were mixed with equal amounts of Freund's complete adjuvant (Difco) and used as antigen. Two intramuscular injections spaced by 5 weeks were given and blood drawn one week after the second injection. The bovine antiserum had a neutralising antibody titre above 1:30,000 and was used to produce fluorescein-labelled antibody (Beutner et al., 1968).

A bovine antiserum to goat IgG was produced by giving a 6-month-old calf a series of intramuscular injections of an 8% solution of goat IgG in Freund's complete adjuvant. The injections (3 ml) were given at intervals of 2 weeks and after the sixth injection serum was collected and used for preparation of antibodies for conjugation with peroxidase (Sigma Chemical Co. type IV) using the periodate method as described elsewhere (Boorsma and Streefkerk, 1979). The bovine antibodies to goat IgG were isolated on an immunoadsorbent of goat Ig immobilised (Harboe and Ingild, 1973) on glutaraldehyde activated Ultrogel AcA 22 (Reactifs IBF-Pharmindustrie - France). The immunosorbent Ultrogel AcA 22 was prepared according to the instructions of the manufacturer. The bovine antibodies in goat IgG were eluted from the immunoadsorbent using a 0.1 M glycine buffer pH 2.3.

Demonstration of BVD virus by PO staining

Ten μl of each serum were dispensed into each of 4 wells in a 96-well flat-bottom microtitre plate. To 2 of these wells were then added 50 μl of Eagle's MEM with 5% calf serum. To the 2 other wells, serving as controls, was added the same amount of medium containing the bovine anti-BVD hyperimmune serum in a final dilution of 1:200. After incubation at room temperature for 1 h, 0.1 ml of a suspension containing about 2×10^5/ml BK 347 cells was added to each well. The plate was covered by a lid and incubated in a humidified atmosphere with 5% CO_2 for 4 days at 37°C. The cells were then fixed in 20% acetone in PBS containing 0.4% calf serum. To fix the cells better to the bottom of the wells, the plates were dried for 3 hours in the incubator at 37°C. Staining was accomplished by adding 0.05 ml of a 1:200 dilution of the goat anti-BVD virus serum to each well and after 30 mins. and 4 washings a 1:200 dilution of peroxidase-conjugated bovine antibodies to goat IgG was added and allowed to react for 30 mins. It was essential to add both fixative and the reagents in subsequent steps cautiously to avoid loosing the cell layer. The substrate was 10 μl 30% H_2O_2 in a freshly prepared solution consisting of 8 ml 3-amino-9-ethyl-carbazole dissolved first in 1.2 ml N,N dimethylformamide then in 20 ml 0.05 M acetate buffer pH 5.0. Before addition of the substrate the plates were washed twice in the acetate buffer (Jensen, 1981).

Demonstration of BVD virus in serum samples by FA staining

One hundred μl amounts of serum were dispensed into the wells of

4-well tissue culture plates with a 12 mm circular coverslip deposited in each well. To each well was then added 1 ml of a suspension CT cells (2nd-10th passage) containing about 10^5 cells/ml, and the plates were incubated as described above. The cells were fixed in 80% acetone. Washing, staining with fluorescein-conjugated bovine anti-BVD serum, and mounting in buffered glycerine followed standard procedures.

Serum neutralisation test

The test was carried out as a microtitre test (Frey and Liess,1971). The strongly cytopathogenic BVD virus strain VD 133 was used as the test strain.

RESULTS

Because BVD virus replicates in the leucocytes of infected animals, buffy coat preparations are usually used as a source of virus for detection of BVD. However, when results of virus isolation from buffy coat preparations and serum of clotted samples drawn from animals in the acute stage of an experimental infection were compared it was found that serum was at least as good a source of virus as washed leucocytes in the antibody-free animal (Table 1).

TABLE 1 Isolation and demonstration by FA of BVD virus from buffy coat and serum from 8 calves experimentally infected by intranasal/oral inoculation with two strains of BVD virus. Serum and EDTA-stabilised samples collected 0-11 days pi.

Buffy coat	- ve	+ ve	+ ve	- ve
serum	- ve	- ve	+ ve	+ ve
Calf 1	7	1	3	1
2	6	1	4	1
3	6	1	4	1
4	6	1	4	1
5	7	1	3	1
6	11	0	0	1
7	11	0	0	1
8	11	0	1	0
Total	65	5	19	7

The PO technique described in this report was primarily designed to detect BVD virus in bovine sera. Therefore due considerations had to be given to possible sources of non-specific staining that might interfere with the test. The indirect staining technique using a goat hyperimmune serum to BVD virus and peroxidase-conjugated immunopurified bovine antibodies to goat Ig gave very clear-cut staining reactions of the infected cells. Direct staining of the cells with either caprine or bovine PO-conjugated anti-BVD virus Ig was found to be less satisfactory because rather low dilutions of conjugate were necessary to get clear-cut staining.

BVD virus isolates from serum samples are usually non-cytopathogenic and in most cases all the cells in the wells are infected when samples from clinical cases of BVD are tested. Although the reactions of such samples may be detected macroscopically it is necessary to examine the plates by low-power microscopy to reveal single infected cells or infected foci. When the samples were examined by both FA and PO techniques the cultures stained by the PO-technique appeared to be more heavily infected.

Non-specific staining occasionally occurred when samples were heavily contaminated with bacteria, but in such cases the control wells were stained with equal intensity.

The indirect PO staining for BVD virus in microtitre plates was found to be more sensitive than FA staining of cultures grown in 24-well tissue culture plates. When the same 132 diagnostic samples were examined by both techniques, agreement of results were found in 126 (95%) of the cases. Of these, 53 were positive and 73 negative for BVD virus by both techniques. The PO technique detected BVD virus in 5 samples that were found negative by FA, and the FA technique revealed one sample that had been negative by the PO technique.

SN antibody-free diagnostic samples that were found negative for BVD virus by the PO staining were passaged in 24-well plates, and after freezing supernatants were tested by PO staining in microtitre plates. Of the 462 samples positive for BVD virus (Table 2), 455 (98%) were positive without a second passage.

Table 2 summarises the results of PO staining for BVD virus performed on sera from healthy and clinically affected cattle. The samples from the 2 slaughterhouses comprised only adult animals. The results illustrate the widespread occurrence of the infection, in that 78% were antibody carriers and 0.9% were viremic.

TABLE 2   BVD virus infections: Neutralising antibody and BVD
           virus in sera from healthy and clinically affected
           cattle.

	Total (%)	SN-ab pos ($\geqslant$1:4)		SN-ab neg ($<$ 1:4)	
		virus +	virus −	virus +	virus −
Apparently healthy cattle (slaughter-house)	1332(100)	0	1042(78)	12(0.9)	278(22)
Apparently healthy cattle from 13 herds with recent outbreaks of BVD	363(100)	0	317(87)	38(10.5)	8(2.5)
Diagnostic samples from animals suspected of BVD	1313(100)	7(0.5)	613(47)	462(35)	231(18)

In herds that had experienced recent losses from BVD an average of
13% of animals were serologically negative, and 38 (83%) of 46 seronegative animals were viremic. According to information from practising
veterinarians, the majority of these animals appeared healthy at the time
of the sampling. As the purpose of the laboratory examination in these
cases was to find the non-immune animals in order to limit losses in the
herds, seronegative animals were slaughtered and could therefore not be
studied further.

Of the 469 diagnostic samples that carried BVD virus, 7 were found to
have low levels of neutralising antibodies (1:4 - 1:5.6) to the test strain.
This finding may reflect the serological heterogeneity of BVD virus also
reported by others (Maisonnave and Rossi, 1982).

To see whether the difference in clinical condition was reflected in
the amount of virus in the blood, the blood distribution of BVD virus
titres in the serum of 70 apparently healthy animals and the same number of
animals with clinical disease were compared (Fig. 1). In animals with
clinical disease, titres as high as $10^{5.5}$ TCID$_{50}$/0.01 ml were found, but
there is only a slight significant difference between the means of the two
groups (2.6 and 3.1). In persistently infected animals, BVD virus titres
in serum seem to be rather constant over long periods of time. One animal
has been followed for more than a year, one animal for 7 months. Both
animals appear healthy (Fig. 2).

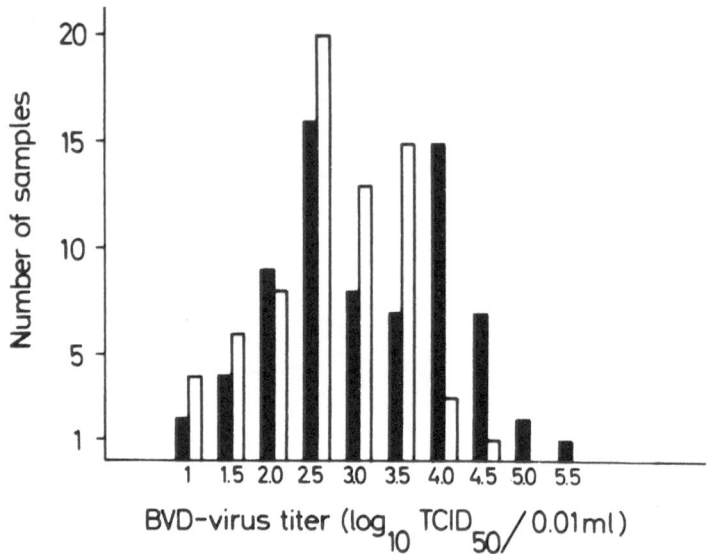

Fig.1   Distribution of BVD virus titres in serum from viremic cattle.
Clinically affected animals, solid bars, mean titre $10^{3.1}$
$TCID_{50}/0.01$ ml. Apparently healthy, cattle open bars, mean
titre $10^{2.6}$ $TCID_{50}/0.01$ ml. (t 2.74, p< 0.01). End points
determined by PO staining.

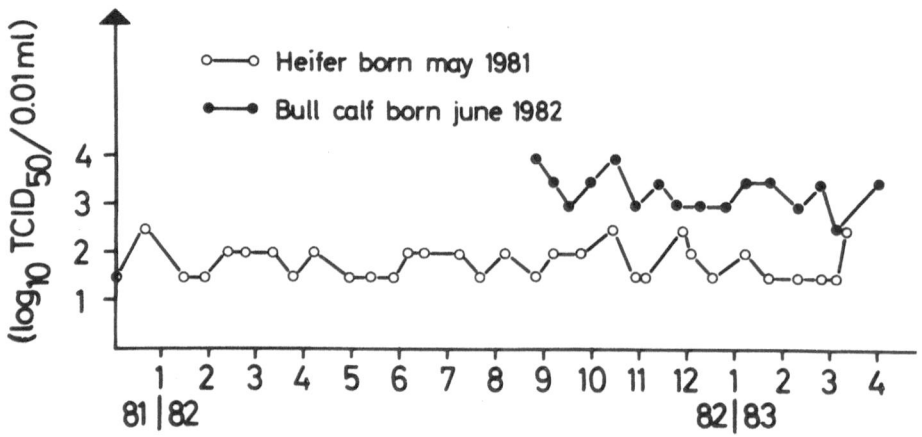

Fig. 2   BVD virus titres in serum of persistently infected animals.
End points determined by PO staining.

DISCUSSION

The PO technique described here is relatively simple provided the necessary antisera for producing the reagents are at hand. Once the test conditions have been established, the procedure is much easier to perform and read than other tests described for detection and identification of non-cytopathogenic BVD virus.

The observations on the antibody prevalence reported in this paper are in agreement with earlier work and with results reported from other countries (Dinter and Borgen, 1964; Harkness et al., 1978). The use of PO staining has made virus isolation and titration manageable even with large number of samples and this study revealed that as many as 0.9% of adult animals brought to slaughter were viremic. It was not established how and when these animals became infected, but it seems reasonable to assume that the majority were persistently infected. In herds that had experienced losses due to BVD, only 13% of the remaining animals were seronegative and 83% of these were found to be viremic. This finding implies that vaccination would have little or no immediate effect on the mortality in such herds.

A simple technique like PO staining for detection of BVD virus is of practical importance, since viremic animals from herds that have had fatal cases of BVD constitute a special risk group with high mortality. Losses in such herds may be reduced if the viremic animals are sold for slaughter before they get the clinical disease. Some persistently viremic animals may live and appear to be healthy for years, and even breed. These animals constantly excrete virus from external secretions and therefore represent a source of infection (Coria and McClurkin, 1978). The technique described is well suited to diagnose this condition.

REFERENCES

Beutner, E.H., Sepulveda, Marion, R. and Bernett, E.V. (1968). Quantitative studies of immunofluorescent staining. Bull. Wld. Hlth. Org., 39, 587-606.
Boorsma, D.M. and Streefkerk, J.G. 1979. Periodate or glutaraldehyde for preparing peroxidase conjugates. J. Immunol. Methods, 20, 245-255.
Coria, M.F. and McClurkin, A.W. 1978. Specific immune tolerance in an apparently healthy bull persistently infected with bovine viral diarrhoea virus. J.A.V.M.A., 172, 449-451.
Dinter, Z. and Borgen, H.C. 1964. Bovine virus diarrhoea (Mucosal Disease) virus in Swedish and Danish Cattle. Nord. Vet. Med., 16, 384-389.
Frey, H.-R. and Liess, B. 1971. Vermehrungskinetik und Verwendbarkeit eines stark zytopathogenen VD-MD-Virusstamme fur diagnostische Untersuchungen mit der Mikrotiter-Methode. Zbl. Vet. Med. B., 18,

61-71.

Gillespie, J.H., Madin, S.H. and Darby, N.B. 1962. Cellular resistance in tissue culture induced by non-cytopathic strains, to a cytopathogenic strain of bovine viral diarrhoea virus of cattle. Proc. Soc. exp. Biol. Med., 110, 248-250.

Harboe, N. and Ingild, A. 1973. Immunization, isolation of immunoglobulins, estimation of antibody titre. Scand. J. Immunol., 2 (suppl. 1), 161-164.

Harkness, J.W., Sands, J.J. and Richards, M.S. 1978. Serological studies of mucosal disease virus in England and Wales. Res. Vet. Sci., 24, 98-103.

Jensen, M.H. 1981. Detection of antibodies against hog cholera virus and bovine viral diarrhoea virus in porcine serum. Acta. Vet. Scand., 22, 85-98.

Maisonnave, J. and Rossi, C.R. 1982. A microtitre test for detection and titrating non-cytopathogenic bovine viral diarrhoea virus. Arch. Virol., 72, 279-287.

Ohmann, H.B. 1983. Pathogenesis of bovine viral diarrhoea - mucosal disease: distribution and significance of BVD-antigen in diseased calves. Res. Vet. Sci., 34, 5-10.

Saunders, G.C. 1977. Development and evaluation of an enzyme-labelled antibody test for rapid detection of hog cholera antibodies. Am. J. Vet. Res., 38, 21-25.

Steck, F., Lazary, S., Wandeler, A., Huggler, Chr., Oppliger, G., Baumberger, H., Karderli, R. and Martig, J. 1980. Immune responsiveness in cattle fatally affected by bovine virus diarrhoea-mucosal disease. Zbl. Vet. Med. B., 27, 429-445.

VIRAL DIAGNOSIS BY ELECTRON MICROSCOPY

June D. Almeida

The Wellcome Research Laboratories
Langley Court
Beckenham, Kent BR3 3BS England

ABSTRACT

The electron microscope (EM) technique of negative staining has become an increasingly useful tool in the viral diagnostic field not only for reaching a primary diagnosis but also for corroborating the findings produced by more recent techniques. In carrying out negative staining attention to detail is important and this is discussed. The areas where negative staining can be most meaningfully employed are considered and three are delineated. These are, one, where no test based on serology exists, two, where the specimen has an unknown aetiology, and finally, in order to establish a diagnosis with problem specimens. Examples of each of these categories are given and illustrations provided.

Viral diagnosis is a rapidly advancing area within the general field of microbiology and, like many situations where there is rapid progress, uneven development can occur. One laboratory will be using the time honoured techniques of complement fixation and haemagglutination while their neighbours down the road are employing enzyme linked immunosorbent assays (ELISA) and DNA probes. Within this framework there is a need for reference techniques that will give reproducible results and which will act as a yardstick for both established and modern methods. The electron microscope (EM) technique of negative staining which appeared as a method of rapid virus diagnosis in the early 1960s, remains as one of the best of these techniques as it can be used to establish a definitive result in its own right and also to corroborate the results obtained by other methods.

As will be discussed later, consideration of technical detail is all important in carrying out virus diagnosis by the negative staining method and a broad outline of the method is given here (Almeida, 1980).

Clinical Specimen

Almost any type of clinical material will yield a preparation that can be examined by the EM although some will be easier to handle than others. Basically, it is necessary to produce a suspension of virus-containing fluid that can be mixed with negative stain. The suspension should contain no inorganic material such as sodium chloride that will dry out to give crystals and should contain as little low molecular weight protein as possible as this overlays and obscures particles of interest. If the specimen is fluid or semi-solid this can be achieved very simply by making a 10% suspension of specimen in either phosphate buffered saline (PBS) or distilled water and centrifuging at a speed that will precipitate at least some of the virus but will leave low molecular weight material in the supernatant. Diarrhoeal faeces belong in this group and the procedure used in our laboratory is as follows. Approximately 0.1 ml of faecal material is diluted to 1 ml with distilled water in a screw-capped clinical centrifuge tube. This is mixed using a rotary-type mixer and allowed to stand in a rack so that heavy debris settles out. 500 µl of supernatant is then transferred to another tube and centrifuged for one hour at 15,000 g, the supernatant is discarded and the tube thoroughly drained by putting it into a beaker with the open end down. However, while 500 µl of faecal suspension is usually available, other types of specimen may have much less material for examination. In these instances as little as 50 µl can be used although for ease of handling this can be diluted tenfold with PBS for centrifugation. Solid tissue is prepared for EM by once again making a 10% suspension, this time using a suitable homogeniser such as one of the Tenbroek type. Fluid specimens such as serum, urine, or tissue culture supernatant need only be centrifuged for the hour at 15,000 g although if there is high level of protein, as in serum, the specimen should be diluted 1/10 in distilled water before centrifugation to give a cleaner specimen. Usually more than one specimen will be examined at a time and the beaker containing inverted tubes is used to transport the specimens to the EM laboratory if it is separate from the main virus laboratory.

The point about draining tubes after centrifugation is the one mentioned earlier about getting rid of both inorganic salts and low molecular weight material. It should also be remarked that the relatively low speed used for centrifugation is an attempt to strike a balance between virus recovery on the one hand and avoidance of too much contaminating low molecular weight protein on the other.

The pellet obtained from this preparatory operation is now ready for negative staining.

Grids

Electron microscope grids come in a range of mesh sizes and forms for different specialist purposes. Since negative staining yields specimens that contain a wide range of three dimensional structures, they put considerable stress on the substrate and therefore only small mesh grids with a stable supporting film should be used. 400 mesh copper grids with a carbon-formvar film are most widely employed.

Negative Stain

Although a wide range of negative stains exist the original phosphotungstic acid remains a widely used reagent (Haschemeyer and Myers, 1972). For ordinary purposes it is used as a 3% or 4% solution in triple distilled water adjusted to pH6 with 1N KOH. However it should be remembered that some viruses, particularly rhinoviruses and foot and mouth disease virus, are pH labile and require stain adjusted to pH8.

Method of preparing grid

The specimen tube, which till now has remained inverted, is examined for the presence of any residual fluid. This can be removed with a strip of filter paper, remembering however, that the fluid could contain infectious virus. The tube is then turned right way up and approximately 50 μl of distilled water added by a Pasteur pipette. The same pipette is then used to resuspend the pellet which in some specimens, for example faeces, will be large, while in others, such as tissue culture supernatants, may not even be visible. A small aliquot of this suspension is placed on a microscope slide and adjusted to a suitable dilution with more distilled water. In the case of the specimen which did not yield a visible pellet no further dilution is made while the thick faecal suspension has more distilled water added until the suspension is only just opalescent. An equal quantity of 4% phosphotunstic acid (PTA) is added to the final dilution and, after mixing, a drop is placed on a prepared grid. Excess fluid is withdrawn with filter paper and the grid is left to dry for a few minutes at which time it is ready for examination in the microscope.

This procedure has the advantage that the centrifugation step both concentrates the virus and at the same time allows low molecular weight material to be discarded. However, if there is a particular need to provide a very rapid result it is possible to carry out an 'on the grid' method that can be accomplished in a matter of minutes. The specimen must be fluid or semi-fluid, eg tissue culture suspension, allantoic fluid, or faeces, if not, a homogenised suspension must be made. A drop of specimen is diluted on the slide with distilled water until the suspension is only just turbid. A drop of this mixture is then placed on a forceps-held grid and, after allowing a few seconds for adsorption, excess fluid is withdrawn and the grid is washed by gently dropping distilled water onto it. Distilled water is then replaced with 2% PTA and final excess fluid withdrawn with filter paper. The grid is allowed to dry and is ready for examination in the microscope. This method takes only a few minutes to carry out but relies on initial virus titre and, because low molecular weight material is able to attach to the carbon-formvar, it gives a less clear picture. In spite of this, it is a method that can be useful for the examination of several specimen types, particularly vesicle fluid and faeces, and gives results only a little less sensitive than the centrifugation method.

If the 'on the grid' method is a little less sensitive than the standard centrifugation method then immune electron microscopy (IEM) is rather more sensitive. The principle of this method is that, in the presence of antiserum, virus is clumped into immune aggregates. These complexes are more efficiently recovered from the centrifugation step and are also more readily visualised in the EM. Together, these factors mean that the specimen can be screened at a lower magnification than when there are only individual particles, in turn this means that there is a better sampling effect with subsequent improvement in sensitivity. In practice IEM has been the first method to characterise several viruses of importance (Kapikian et al., 1972; Feinstone et al., 1973).

IEM is carried out in exactly the same manner as for standard negative staining except that the original virus-containing specimen suspension is allowed to react with a suitable amount of antiserum. The antiserum employed can be of two types, first, a specific antiserum raised for the purpose when the virus of interest is known. An example of this category would be rotavirus for which good antisera are available and where epidemiological studies are of importance. Secondly, when the virus is uncharacterised, a recovery serum from either the same animal or a member of the same flock or herd can be used. A variant of this approach is the use of 'old cow' serum on the basis that a mature animal will have been exposed to most of the circulating pathogens and is likely to have antibodies to them. Whichever serum type is employed it is necessary to add it to the virus suspension at a level to give good complex formation.

Usually, the suitable range for a serum is wide, and often all that is required with an unknown serum is to use it at a 1/10 and a 1/100 dilution
on the first occasion of use. A suitable dilution, that may be intermediate between 1/10 and 1/100 or occasionally an even greater dilution can
then be established. Many sera are satisfactory at 1/50 which will give
complex formation with both high and low titre virus preparations. Virus
suspension and antiserum are left to react for two hours at room temperature or overnight at 4°C. After this step the mixture is treated exactly
as for the simple virus suspension. In a situation of urgency the virus
antibody mixture can be incubated at 37°C for 30 mins before centrifugation.

Interpretation

Negative staining is an efficient means of virus diagnosis because of
two facts. The first is that viruses, for the most part, have an unmis-
takable appearance, with the best, but not all displaying distinctive geometric subunits. The second is that, because the stain of negative staining is applied around the particle, there is build up of electron dense
material surrounding the virus more than around cell debris. This means
that virus is highlighted by a dark surrounding halo while other structures
show less contrast and appear in shades of grey (Fig. 1). These two facts
are themselves related as the build up of stain around the particles is
due to the virus having a more three dimensional form than the surrounding
cell fragments. However, in spite of this, difficulties still arise with
some of the membrane bound viruses when identification relies on surface
projections. Coronaviruses in particular are difficult as some cell components for example, mitichondria, also have surface projections. However,
if technically good specimens are produced this should not be a serious
problem as each type of projection is distinctive, and form can be used to
distinguish viral from cellular components (Almeida, 1983).

Sensitivity

A recent study, to be reported elsewhere, of several hundred faecal
samples examined by both Elisa and EM has shown that if both tests are
carried out optimally then they have an equal sensitivity. However, it is
obvious that sensitivity is not an isolated factor but is related to specimen type and virus type. The detection of a beautifully geometric adenovirus in a thin diarrhoeal suspension is an easy task while a non-

distinctive arbovirus in a spleen homogenate will be much more difficult. The pertinent factor can be described as the ratio of signal to noise and this will influence tests other than electron microscopy, so that it probably remains correct that EM and more particularly IEM has a sensitivity similar to that of the enzyme conjugated assays but rather less than that of radioimmunoassay.

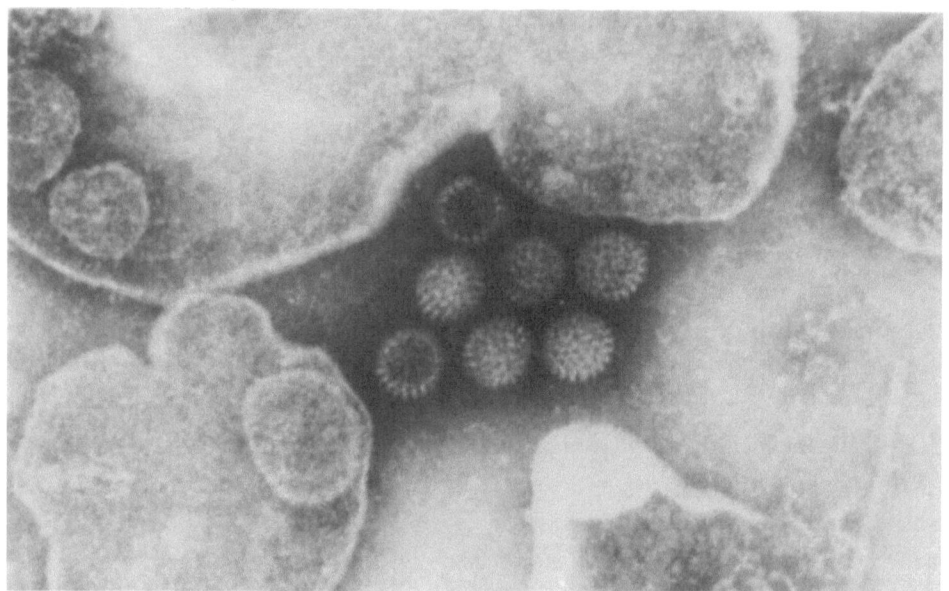

Fig. 1   A group of rotavirus particles present in a faecal specimen. Although there is considerable debris surrounding the virus they stand out because of the dense rim of negative stain and their own geometric construction.   Mag. X180,000.

In absolute terms, the EM is capable of detecting virus at a level somewhere between 10^5 and 10^6 particles per ml of starting material. However, in some instances, better sensitivity will be obtained as the microscope is capable of recognising viral components as well as complete virus. An illustration of this is shown further on (Fig. 4b). Another method of increasing the sensitivity of the EM is to use it as a secondary technique, using a primary growth in tissue culture with subsequent examination of the in-vitro grown material. Although not as rapid as direct examination, this approach can nevertheless save much time, as a diagnosis of virus type, at least, can frequently be made after an overnight growth step followed by EM examination on the next morning.

False Negatives

Any technique not based on the rescue of live virus must theoretically give rise to false negatives as the numbers of particles necessary for any serological or observational method will be greater than that needed for virus growth. In addition to these general considerations there is also the question of variation between laboratories. In a study of faecal specimens it was found that while one EM laboratory made 8 out of 22 specimens positive another group found only three positives among the same specimens. This finding is not surprising as poor EM results are encountered all too frequently. In almost every case they are caused by inappropriate preparatory technique. This will be discussed in the technical problems section.

False Positives

Unlike techniques based on the mass serological action of virus, the EM makes its finding by direct visualisation of individual virus particles. This means that false positive results should theoretically never occur.

Unfortunately they do, but they are mediated by contamination rather than a spurious cross reaction. The commonest means of contaminating an EM specimen is by the forceps used to hold the grid. Small amounts of fluid run onto the legs of the forceps, dry out, and are later resuspended by a subsequent specimen. The best means of ridding the forceps of virus is by flaming, a method which does not prolong the life of the forceps but is the only technique that can be trusted.

Technical Problems

Many false negatives occur because the specimen has been centrifuged for too long at too high a g force. A recent publication which will not be quoted, compared Elisa with EM and found electron microscopy a very poor second. However, all specimens for EM had been centrifuged for 2 hours at 100,000 g. After such treatment any virus which had not been permanently impacted into the tube wall would be buried beneath a carpet of the low molecular weight material which is brought down at this speed. To illustrate how little centrifugation is needed to produce an acceptable specimen a rotavirus IEM preparation was prepared by centrifuging it in a bench centrifuge and the pellet used for negative staining. The force employed was approximately 2000 g yet this was sufficient to yield a

54

positive result with both aggregated and single particles present (Fig. 2).

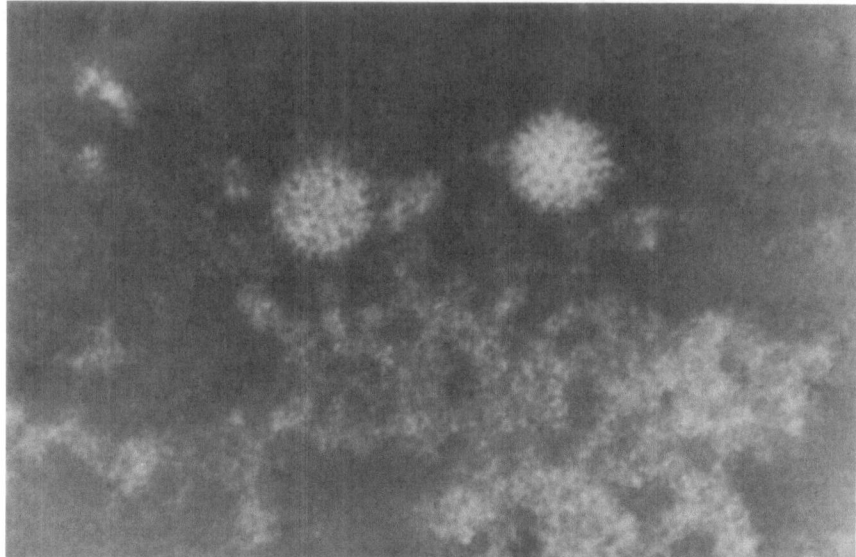

Fig. 2   Virus can be recovered from specimens even when centrifuged
at very low g force. This specimen was spun at only 2000 g and
although background debris is present the rotavirus has been clearly
resolved. Mag. X180,000.

The second crucial preparation point is the amount of material in the
distilled water suspension of the virus containing pellet. A common fault
of the beginner is to make this suspension too thick, the fear being that
if it is almost clear there cannot possibly be enough virus for visualisation. It is worth remembering that, unless the specimen contains more
than 10^{12} particles/ml the actual virus will not contribute to the overall
opacity of the specimen. What is being seen is the background material
that, if present in too high concentration, will obscure any virus present.
It is therefore important to produce a specimen where even the smallest
virus (Fig. 3) can be seen against a relatively clear background, and this
can only be done when the starting suspension is no more than slightly
opalescent.

Disadvantages of Negative Staining
There are two major drawbacks to using the EM for virus diagnosis.
First the initial outlay for an electron microscope, and second the fact
that it is a work intensive technique calling for a certain degree of ex-
pertise. In spite of the high cost of the equipment most virology

laboratories now have, or have access to, an EM so this problem does not seem to be unsurmountable. The second problem can best be dealt with by ensuring that the EM is used only for those categories of specimen which cannot be tested more efficiently by other techniques, and this will be discussed in the next section.

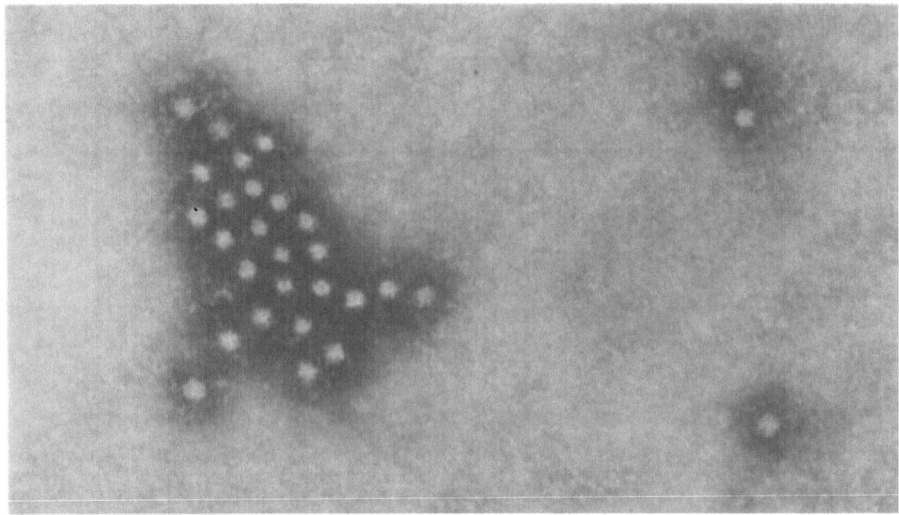

Fig. 3   This micrograph shows the satellite virus of infectious bursal disease and although it is only 18 nm in diameter both it and the attached antibody can be well resolved when low molecular weight material is excluded.   Mag. X180,000.

Application of Negative Staining

If one considers the recent past it can be seen that the EM was fre-quently the first technique by which a virus or antigen was first detected. For example, the particulate nature of hepatitis B antigen was recognised in negatively stained specimens of serum (Bayer et al., 1968), and the existance of a new virus group, the Rotaviridae was established by EM (Flewett et al., 1974).   In both these instances, for the period immediate-ly following their discovery, the EM was the only available means of de-tection.   However, within a short space of time immunoassays were developed for the detection of both HBAg and rotavirus (Lander et al., 1971; Kapikian et al., 1974).   It would now be ridiculous to consider screening routine blood donations for the presence of hepatitis B antigen by EM and, similarly, an epidemiological survey of faecal samples for rotavirus would be a very wasteful use of an electron microscope.   Straightforward radio-immunoassays and Elisa assays can be carried out on large numbers of both specimen types with a minimum of work input related to results of high sensitivity and specificity. However, the situation reverses if, instead of a large number of specimens, one individual specimen or a small number of specimens, have to be tested accurately and quickly. For example, if one calf scours in an otherwise clean herd, it is important to establish quickly whether virus or bacteria are implicated. A quick EM examination will establish not only if rotavirus is present but whether any other recognisable viral agent is present. The point here is that, while an immunoassay must be directed to a specific virus the EM scans for virus in general rather than one virus in particular.

This ability to recognise any virus that is present rather than the one that is being detected by an immunoassay leads to the second group of specimens suitable for EM. These are those with no known aetiological agent. Immunoassays are not suitable for this group and the only alternative to direct visualisation is by isolation on tissue culture which can be a long, tedious, and not always successful undertaking. Two examples of this type of specimen are illustrated here. Fig. 4a shows the morphological appearance of a virus that was present in the lungs of marmosets dying from a respiratory disease that had affected the colony. Full diagnosis actually took two steps. A rapid EM examination showed a virus belonging to the paramyxoviridae family and immunofluorescence identified it as a parainfluenza I virus (Gardner, this volume). The marmoset lung specimen also illustrates the ability of the EM to identify viral components as well as whole virus. Fig. 4b shows a large quantity of helical internal component (RNP) that is diagnostic of paramyxoviridae and which would have been recognised even if present in much lower amount.

A second example of this type of 'one off' situation is illustrated by the finding of an adenovirus in guinea pig lung (Fig. 5). Once again as for the marmosets, the guinea pig colony had developed an outbreak of respiratory disease that could not be shown to have a bacterial origin. Direct examination of lung homogenate revealed the presence of large numbers of adenovirus particles and later tests by IEM showed that affected animals had seroconverted to this virus. Together, these findings established that the adenovirus was the cause of the problem.

The third category that is well dealt with by EM is the problem specimen. There are many reasons why a specimen can become a problem but among the more obvious are the following. A specimen gives a negative result

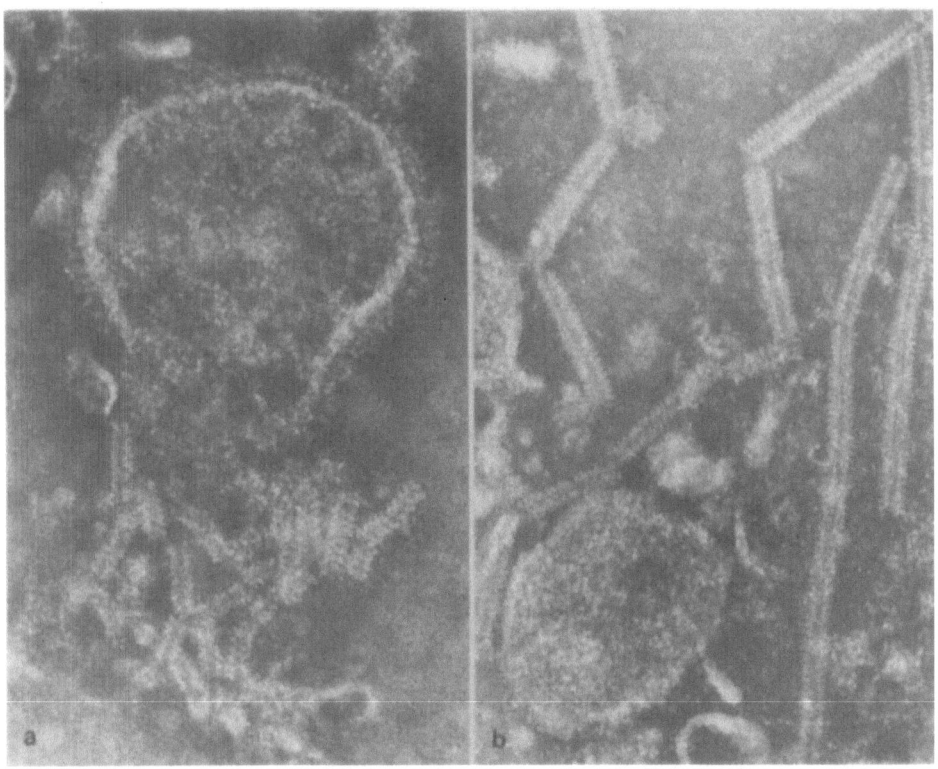

Fig. 4a   The EM is an important diagnostic tool for specimens with
no known aetiological agent. This figure shows a parainfluenza
virus that was detected by direct visualisation in the lungs of
marmosets with respiratory disease. Mag. X180,000.

Fig. 4b   One of the strengths of the EM is that it can detect viral
components as well as complete virus. This micrograph is from the
same specimen as is shown in Fig. 4a and illustrates the large amount
of RNP that was present. Mag. X180,000.

when all the field data suggests that it should be positive. A specimen
reads positive in one laboratory and negative in another. A variant of
this is when a specimen is positive by one type of test and negative by
another. Whatever the reason, the EM, because it provides photographic
evidence to back up its findings, is frequently able to establish a diagnosis in the face of conflicting findings. For example, the accompanying
micrograph (Fig. 6) is from a sample that was positive in one ELISA test
for rotavirus but not in another. As can be seen, a virus was present but
it is an adenovirus and one must presume that in the case of the test giving a positive rotavirus result the antiserum employed contained antibody

58

to adenovirus as well as rotavirus.

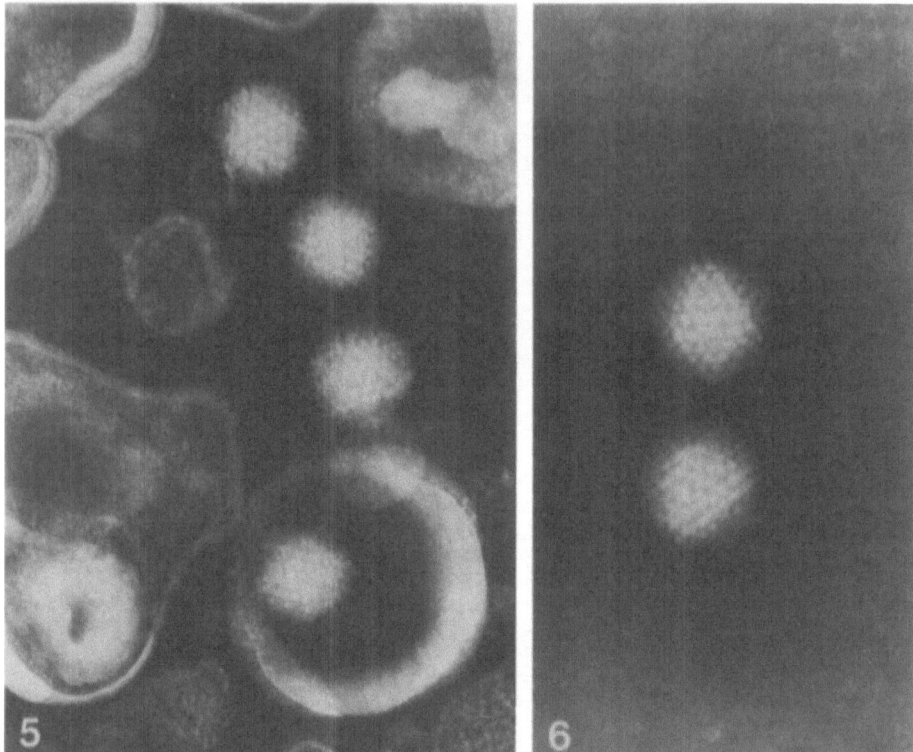

Fig. 5   Guinea pigs with respiratory disease were shown by EM to
have a high titre of adenovirus in lung homogenates. A typical field
with easily recognisable adenovirus is shown here. Mag. X230,000.

Fig. 6   A faecal specimen gave conflicting results with two ELISA
tests for rotavirus. EM showed that the specimen actually contained
adenovirus. Mag. X220,000.

The Future

Since the sensitivity of the EM using the negative staining technique
still equals that of current immunoassay methods, the present technology
will be capable of providing meaningful results at least for the near future. On a longer term basis one could look for improvements in specimen
preparation resulting in an improvement in the recovery of virus in relationship to the amount of background material. Although not yet completely satisfactory there are a number of methods for using the microscope
grid as a solid phase and employing a layer of capture antibody (Goldwater
et al., 1979). This technique is known as solid phase immune electron

microscopy (SPIEM) and developments along this line could lead to improvements both in preparation time and sensitivity (Obert et al., 1981). It could well be that SPIEM in tandem with the use of monoclonal antibodies could lead to a technology where only virus is able to adsorb to the specimen grid. However, until such improvements have occurred the present day EM technique of negative staining with its extension into IEM will yield many useful diagnostic results and resolve some otherwise sticky problems.

REFERENCES

Almeida, J.D. 1980. Practical aspects of diagnostic electron microscopy. Yale J. Biol. Med., 53, 5-18.

Almeida, J.D. 1983. Uses and Abuses of Diagnostic Electron Microscopy. In "Current Topics in Microbiology and Immunology, Vol. 104" (Ed. M. Cooper, P.H. Hofschneider, H. Koprowski, F. Melchers, R. Rott, H.G. Schweiger, P.K. Vogt and R. Zinkernagel). (Springer-Verlag, Berlin Heidelburg). pp. 147-158.

Bayer, M.E., Blumberg, B.S. and Werner, B. 1968. Particles associated with Australia antigen in the sera of patients with leukaemia, Down's syndrome and hepatitis. Nature, 218, 1057.

Feinstone, S.M., Kapikian, A.Z. and Purcell, R.H. 1973. Hepatitis A detection by immune electron microscopy of a virus-like antigen associated with acute illness. Science, 182, 1026-1028.

Flewett, T.H., Davies, H., Bryden, A.S. and Robertson, M.J. 1974. Diagnostic electron microscopy of faeces, II. Acute gastroenteritis associated with reovirus-like particles. J. Clin. Pathol., 27, 603-614.

Goldwater, P.N., Chrystie, I.L. and Banatvala, J.E. 1979. Rotavirus and the respiratory tract. Br. Med. J., 2, 1551.

Haschemeyer, R.H. and Myers, R.J. 1972. Negative Staining. In "Principles and techniques of electron microscopy. Biological applications. Vol.2" (Ed. M.A. Hayat). (van Nostrand Reinhold, New York). pp. 101-147.

Kapikian, A.Z., Wyatt, R.G., Dolin, R., Thornhill, T.S., Kalica, A.R. and Chanock, R.M. 1972. Visualisation by immune electron microscopy of a 27 nm particle associated with acute infectious nonbacterial gastroenteritis. J. Virol., 10, 1075-1081.

Kapikian, A.Z., Kim, H.W., Wyatt, R.G., Rodringuez, W.J., Ross, S., Cline, W.L., Parrott, R.H. and Chanock, R.M. 1974. Reovirus-like agent in stools: association with infantile diarrhoea and development of serologic tests. Science, 185, 1049-1053.

Lander, J.J., Alter, H.J. and Purcell, R.H. 1971. Frequency of antibody to hepatitis-associated antigen as measured by a new radioimmunoassay technique. J. Immunol., 106, 1166-1171.

Obert, G., Gloeckler, R., Burckard, J. and Van Regenmortel, M.H.V. 1981. Comparison of immunosorbant electron microscopy, enzyme immunoassay and counterimmunoelectrophoresis for detection of human rotavirus in stools. J. Virol. Methods, 3, 99-107.

CAPTURE ASSAYS FOR THE DETECTION OF VIRUS-SPECIFIC IgM ANTIBODY

Dr Richard S. Tedder

Department of Virology (Microbiology)
Middlesex Hospital Medical School
School of Pathology
Riding House Street
London W1P 7LD

ABSTRACT

Class-specific antibody capture assays have been developed for a number of human virus infections, in particular for the detection of IgM antibody. These assays, MACRIA's, have a number of advantages over the more conventional indirect solid-phase immunoassays. They are sensitive and unaffected by rheumatoid factor and particularly suited to detecting specific IgM in sera from neonates. While veterinarians will need to develop species-specific anti-µFc antisera, the compensation is that once this is done, the pair of appropriately balanced reagents, virus antigen and its labelled antibody, will be suitable to diagnose recent infection by a given virus in any animal species.

INTRODUCTION

The diagnosis of an acute infection has until recently depended upon either the direct identification of a specific agent or the demonstration of a rise in antibody against that agent. The identification of the infectious agent sometimes relies upon the ability of a laboratory to propagate that agent. But at other times the microbe is not so obliging and its presence has to be demonstrated in other ways, eg by direct microscopy or immunological methods. The alternative of demonstrating a significant rise in antibody titre relies upon the immunological integrity of the host and also requires serum samples taken in the recovery phase of the illness which can be compared with those of the acute phase.

It is particularily this second aspect, the necessity for a late serum, which may limit the usefulness of conventional serological methods in diseases where, for example, environmental control measures may have to be instituted at the earliest opportunity. A similar need for rapid diagnosis in certain human illness, particularily Rubella virus infection (German measles), has led to the development of a new generation of serological assays.

During a primary infection with a virus, the immune system of the host will recognise the presence of the virus and expand the population of those lymphocytes which can both recognise and destroy infected cells by cell-cell interaction and also produce antibodies directed against antigenic components of the virus. Initially, the bulk of the antibody response will be in the IgM class though this will be replaced fairly rapidly by IgG antibody. In some instances therefore it is possible to identify recent infection by detecting a significant amount of virus-specific IgM-class antibody. There are several methods routinely employed for the detection of virus specific IgM antibody. This paper will discuss these but concentrates upon the method known as IgM antibody capture radioimmunoassay (MACRIA).

THE CHOICES

Providing a virus can be grown in vitro, or is available in some quantity from the infected host, it is relatively simple to demonstrate IgM antibody by a number of methods. The reasons for choosing one or other method are generally based on considerations of convenience, cost, sensitivity and specificity - not necessarily ranked in that order.

The most simple methods usually involve solid-phase viral antigen, ie antigen bound either to a plastic surface or fixed in situ in sections of infected tissue. Virus-specific IgM is detected by incubating dilutions of a "patient's" serum over the bound antigen and then measuring the subsequent binding of serum IgM to the solid-phase antigen with a second antibody directed against the Fc portion of the μ chain. The second antibody is usually labelled or tagged with one of a number of indicators, for example fluorescein, colour generating enzymes or radioisotopes (FITC, ELISA or RIA).

Two major problems arise with these types of indirect immunoassay. The first may be due to the relatively low expression of virus antigen in the infected cell or tissue. Much of the solid-phase antigen will be derived from cellular material unrelated to the virus, yet serum IgM may bind to this non-viral component. Though this may be circumvented by careful purification of viral antigen, assays frequently have to incorporate a duplicate solid phase coated with a "control antigen". In addition, if the virus antigen is sparse, then high levels of IgG antibody may prevent binding of low levels of specific IgM. Also, adult sera of humans (and perhaps other species) often contain IgM which has an innate stickiness and which may mask the low level of specific IgM binding.

The second problem arises from the frequent occurrence in sera, particularly from ill hosts, of IgM antibody which reacts with aggregated IgG. This is termed rheumatoid factor (RF) and it is most significant in its ability to give a false-positive reaction in assays for IgM antibody. It does so in the following manner. If a virus is enzootic within a species there will be a high prevalence of immunity. There is a good chance then that any individual will have been infected long before the incident of illness being investigated. Thus sera taken from individuals will frequently contain IgG antibody which will bind specifically to solid-phase antigen. By itself this will not greatly interfere with an assay for IgM antibody although, as mentioned before, it is said that very high levels of IgG may block the binding of specific IgM in some assays. However, in the presence of RF, the IgG bound specifically to antigen will act as a substrate for the RF which, being IgM, will in turn result in a false reaction for specific IgM (Meurman et al., 1977). It is possible to absorb RF from sera giving an IgM reaction by incubation with aggregated IgG before testing for specific IgM. Alternatively, separating the IgM from IgG and re-assaying the IgM fraction in the absence of IgG antibody will prevent the RF from binding to the solid phase.

The principle of separating IgM from IgG antibody introduces the other assays which rely upon certain of the characteristics of M and G class immunoglobulins. The first type of these assays depends upon the physical separation by size of IgM from IgG either by gel filtration or by rate-zonal centrifugation. IgM is a larger molecule than IgG and may be separated quite easily from other immunoglobulins. IgM rich fractions may be tested for antibody, and if they are reactive this may be due to IgM antibody. But, before this reactivity can be designated as virus-specific IgM antibody a number of factors must be considered. In some assays for antibody to viruses such as haemagglutination inhibition or neutralisation, sera may exhibit inhibitory or neutralising substances in the IgM rich fractions which are unrelated to IgM (McFerran et al., 1968). This may be due to lipoprotein and macroglobulins. Further, if a serum has been subjected to repeated freezing and thawing or heat inactivation significant amounts of IgG antibody may be present as aggregates in IgM-rich fractions. For these reasons it is usual to remove non-specific inhibitors before fractionation and to confirm after fractionation that any reactivity is due to IgM by demonstrating its sensitivity to reduction following treatment with 2-Mercaptoethanol (2-ME). Certainly, before consideration is given to the

termination of any human pregnancy on grounds of Rubella virus infection
the final court of appeal should be serum fractionation and demonstration
of reduction - sensitive activity in the IgM fractions (Pattison and Dane,
1975).

Methods relying upon serum fractionation are time consuming and labour
intensive. Consequently, it is not practical for a diagnostic laboratory to
perform more than a small number of such assays each day. Recently tests
for virus-specific IgM have been described which rely upon a different technology, based upon the separation of immunoglobulins on a solid phase coated
with class-specific-antibody to the Fc region of the immunoglobulin molecule. This can be considered as an extension of immune affinity purification and was first described in 1978 (Diament and Pepys, 1978). The
method has achieved wide application in medical diagnostic laboratories and
it is likely that it will also be suitable for veterinarians.

THE PRINCIPLE

In brief, a solid phase is coated with IgG from an anti-serum raised
against μFc. This is then incubated with a dilution of the test serum, IgM
from which is absorbed to the solid phase. After washing, the solid phase
is incubated with a preparation of the relevant viral antigen. If the serum
under test contains significant levels of virus-specific IgM antibody, there
will be increased binding of viral antigen. This can be demonstrated either
by labelling the antigen itself or by demonstrating binding of labelled
antiviral-antibody in a final incubation step using either radiolabelled
antiviral IgG (MACRIA) (Tedder and Wilson-Croome, 1980) or enzyme-labelled
IgG (Gerlich and Luer, 1979). Technically it is easier to develop assays
using a radiolabel.

OPTIMISATION

This will be described by reference to the assay used for detection of
anti-HBc IgM (Tedder and Wilson-Croome, 1980). For any MACRIA there are a
number of steps which have to be optimised. In the case of hepatitis B infections in humans it was not difficult to select a serum from a patient
with hepatitis B which could be expected to contain high levels of specific
IgM antibody to the internal component of the virus. This was confirmed by
fractionation and demonstration of 2-ME-sensitive antibody in the IgM
fraction. Dilutions of this serum and of one negative for all hepatitis B

virus (HBV) markers were incubated overnight over a solid phase coated with sheep anti-human μFc. After washing, the solid phase, in this case poly-styrene tubes, was then incubated with a dilution of HBcAg prepared from the liver of a persistently infected and immunosuppressed patient. After four hours at 37°C, the tubes were washed and ^{125}I anti-HBc, prepared from the serum of a persistently infected patient, incubated in them for a fur-ther 2 hours at 37°C. After a final washing step, the binding of ^{125}I-anti-HBc was measured (Fig. 1). Up to a certain dilution, there is a constant

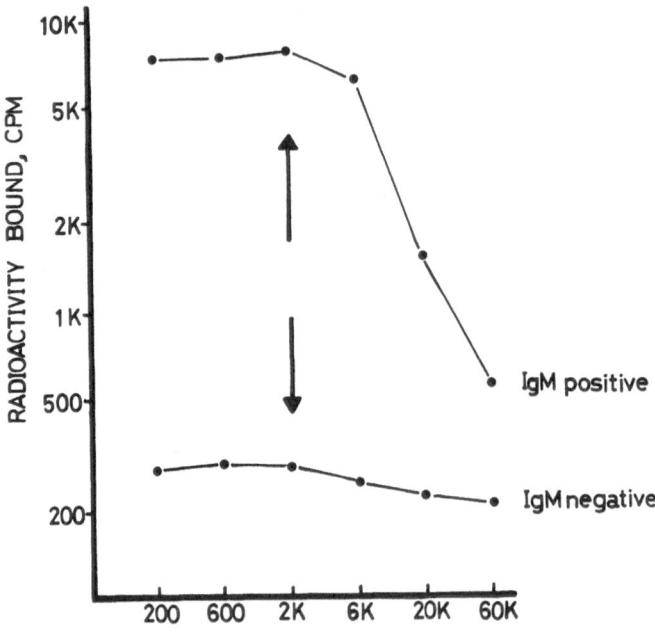

Fig. 1   The effect on binding of ^{125}I-anti-HBc (abscissa) of various dilutions (ordinate) of anti-HBc IgM positive and negative sera. Up to a certain dilution (arrows) the solid phase is saturated with IgM. Beyond this point increasing dilution merely reduced the level of binding displayed by the positive serum.

enhancement of label binding by the IgM-positive serum. The dilution beyond which this enhancement is reduced probably represents that at which the solid phase is no longer saturated with IgM. Some sera containing high levels of specific IgM may cause a prozone at lower dilutions (Fig. 2). A single dilution which avoids the prozone effect should be chosen for the first incubation and it is then possible to construct an assay whereby the

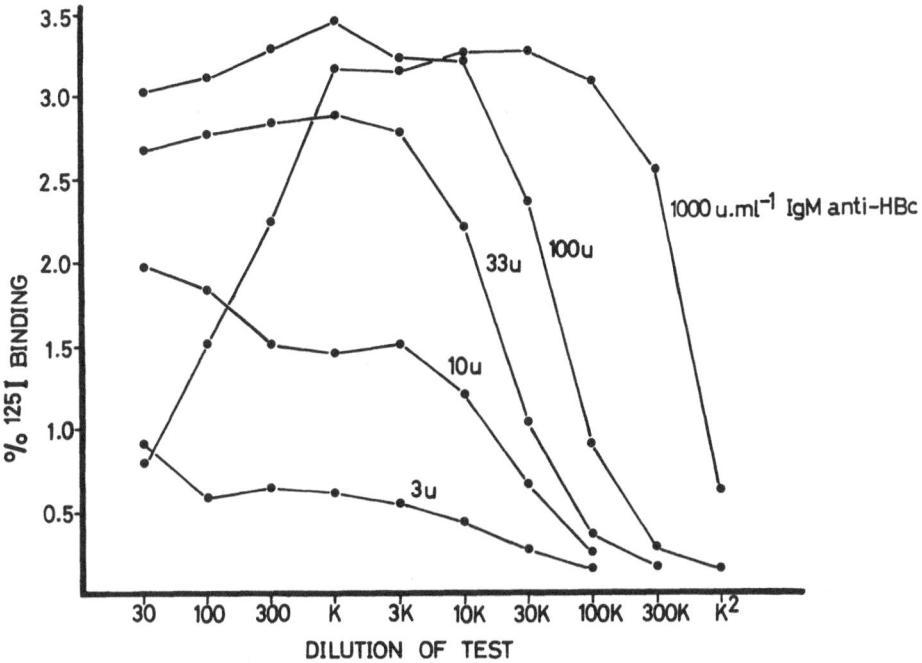

Fig. 2   The effect on binding of ^{125}I-anti-HBc (abscissa) of testing sera containing various levels of anti-HBc IgM (3u/ml up to 1,000 u/ml) at different dilutions in the first step of the test (ordinate). The most highly reactive serum containing 1,000 u/ml exhibited lower binding at dilutions less than 1 in 1000.

more specific IgM contained in a serum the greater the enhancement of ^{125}I-anti-HBc binding (Fig. 3). The fixed dilution will need to be optimised for any particular system and may be markedly different from infection to infection. For example, the MACRIA for hepatitis A IgM is best at a dilution of 1 in 10,000, for hepatitis B anti-HBc IgM at a dilution of 1 in 2,000 and for rubella IgM at a dilution of 1 in 50. The most commonly used diluent is phosphate buffered saline incorporating 0.05% tween 20 or a similar detergent. If sera contain high levels of IgG antibody, as does serum from the human patient persistently infected by HBV, non-specific binding of IgG may be minimised by the addition of protein (0.5% BSA) to the diluent.

Once the dilution of the first stage has been fixed the second and third stages can be optimised. The parameters of the second stage to examine are temperature, time and antigen concentration. Innate stickiness of the antigen may give high background binding which can be suppressed by

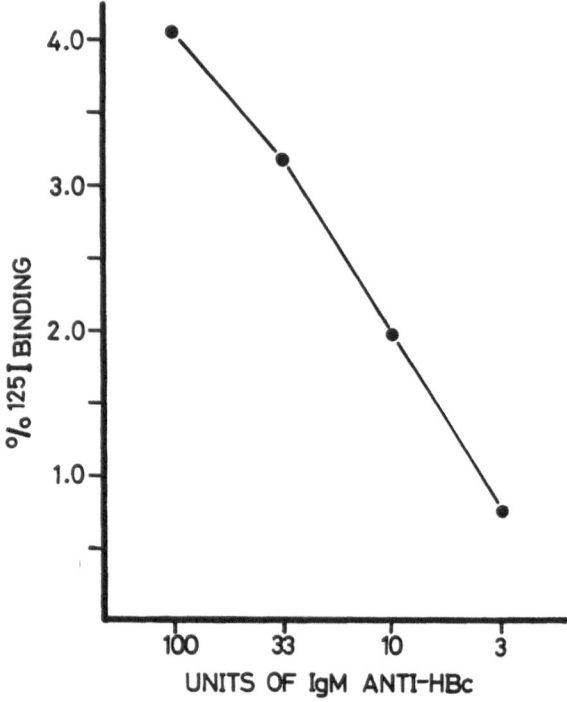

Fig. 3   The effect on binding of ^{125}I-anti-HBc (abscissa) of testing at a single dilution (in this case 1 in 2000) sera containing differing amounts of anti-HBc IgM (3u/ml to 100u/ml, ordinate).

increasing the protein content of the antigen buffer with, for example, foetal calf serum (Sutherland and Briggs, 1983). The final stage can be investigated in a similar manner with time and temperature experiments.

Certain details in the preparation of the labelled IgG are important. It is best to select a serum which has a high level of antibody to the desired viral component. The IgG should be prepared from this by mild conditions, and processes involving high or low pH and salting out should be avoided. Ion exchange chromatography of whole serum is the method of choice. Naturally - occurring high-titre sera can be selected, alternatively a hyperimmune serum may be prepared. However, the advent of monoclonal antibody technology has greatly improved the performance of a number of MACRIAs. The hybridomas are raised against the virus antigen which is to be used in the assay. As a result the narrow specificity of epitope recognition displayed by monoclonal reagents does not present any problem. Nevertheless,

even with a monoclonal reagent, it is best to incorporate into the final
stage buffer sera from all of the various species involved in the assay.
For example in the Rubella MACRIA used in human serology (Tedder et al.,
1982), the final stage diluent includes human serum negative for rubella
antibody and sheep serum, the species in which the anti-μ serum is raised.
Fortunately mouse serum, which is difficult to obtain in quantity, does not
seem to be necessary.

The method used in iodination also affects the performance of the label.
Solid-phase Iodogen (Salacinski et al., 1979) has given the most reliable
and stable labels and results in minimal damage to the antibody. A protein/
iodine ratio of 30 μg per 1mCi ^{125}I is routinely used. Further refinements
can be obtained by passing the labelled protein down a 50 x 1 cm column
packed with Sepharose 6B (Pharmacia Ltd). This serves to remove aggregated
from the monomeric IgG and results in a reduction of the non-specific binding of label. Although not always necessary, this step alone can make the
difference between a test that works and one that doesn't.

SPECIFICITY

Unlike the indirect immunoassay, MACRIA is in normal circumstances unaffected by RF. However, if a serum containing RF and high levels of IgG
antibody is subjected to physical treatment which causes aggregation of
immunoglobulin, it is possible that RF could combine with the aggregated
IgG. If this were to happen, the resulting complex could give a false reaction in MACRIA. In practice, this can only be demonstrated if preformed
aggregates of IgG containing specific antibody are incubated with high-
titre RF. Under these conditions, low levels of reactivity may be generated
(Fig. 4).

There is an additional way in which false-positive reactivity may occur
in both MACRIA and indirect assays. Viruses which bud through membranes may
incorporate into their envelope antigens from the host cells. In some infections, for example primary infection with the Epstein Barr virus, IgM
antibodies against cell glycocalyx antigens may arise. It seems that under
appropriate conditions, these antibodies may bind to a virus antigen which
incorporates cell antigen and give a false positive in MACRIA and in indirect assays (Morgan-Capner et al., 1983). It is important therefore that
before a MACRIA is considered entirely specific, sera from a wide range of
acute infections should be examined to exclude significant false-positive

68

reactivity.

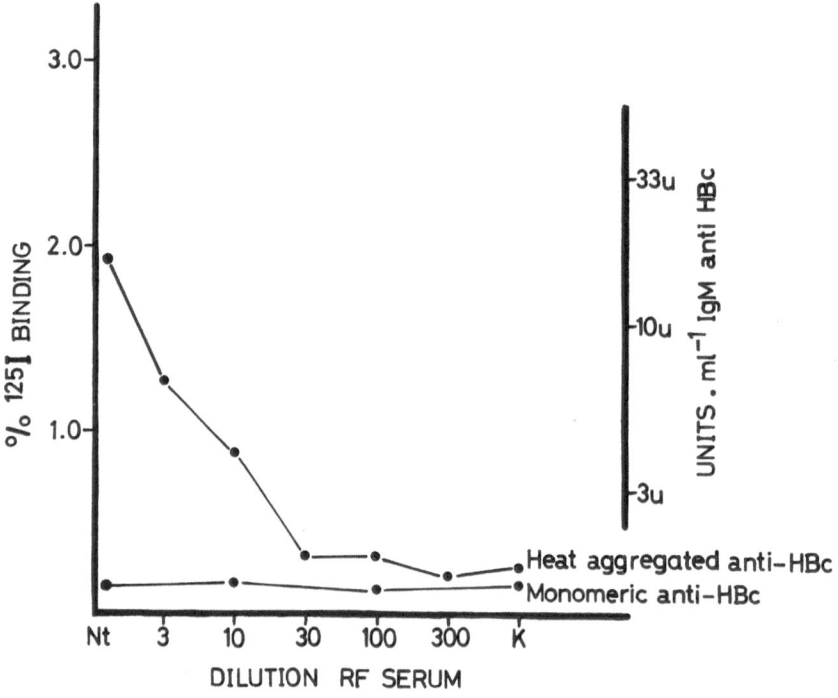

Fig. 4   The effect on binding of ^{125}I-anti-HBc (abscissa) of pre-incubating monomeric or aggregated anti-HBc IgG with various dilutions of RF-positive serum in RF negative serum (ordinate). Following incubation, the serum mixtures were tested in the standard MACRIA for anti-HBc IgM.

QUANTIFICATION

There are two schools of thought concerning quantification of IgM capture assays, either to use the assay as a detector and titrate sera to extinction, or to relate the level of MACRIA reactivity to the level of specific IgM. If an assay has been optimised and strongly reactive sera do not exhibit a prozone, it is possible to perform the test at a single dilution and relate the binding of label to the amount of specific IgM. This is the second option and the more convenient method of the two. Basically, control sera, comprising dilutions in negative serum of a known high titre IgM-positive serum (or pool) given a value in arbitrary units, are measured in each assay. The reactivity of these control sera can be used to construct a calibration curve relating binding of label to units of specific IgM (Fig. 3). Thus, any serum which displays significant reactivity in the test can be ascribed a value for specific IgM in arbitrary units. When a MACRIA is used in this way, the test is in fact measuring the proportion of serum IgM which is specific antibody. This has potential drawbacks. For example, it is possible for two sera having the same MACRIA reactivity to have markedly different levels of total IgM antibody. If a serum contains twice as much specific IgM, but at the same time twice the level of total IgM the proportion of specific to total IgM is the same and so is the MACRIA reactivity. In practice this potential difficulty of using MACRIA to quantify sera at a single dilution does not seem to matter. There is reasonable agreement between anti-HBc IgM levels in sera of patients with acute hepatitis B when measured by MACRIA and by serum fractionation methods (Fig. 5). In situations where the total serum IgM level is low, for

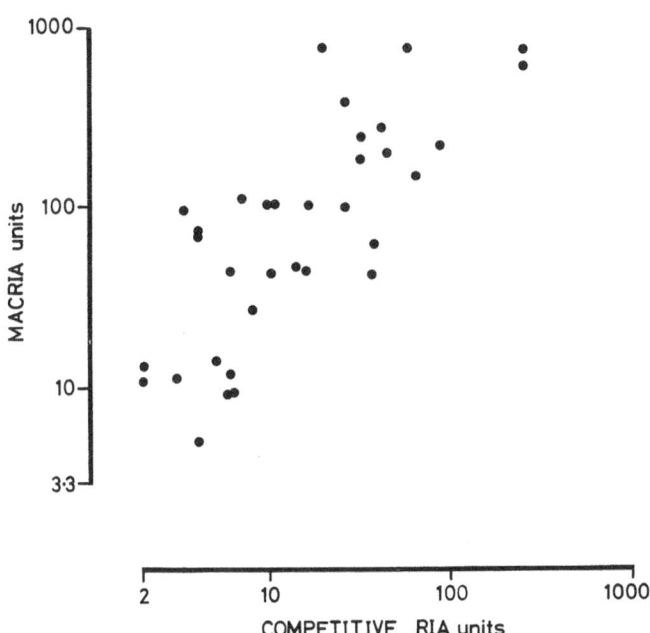

Fig. 5   The relationship between levels of anti-HBc IgM detected in sera from patients with acute hepatitis B measured by MACRIA (abscissa) and by competitive RIA following gel-filtration (ordinate).

example in human neonates, levels of MACRIA reactivity may be greater than expected for low levels of specific IgM. This has an advantage and in fact makes IgM antibody capture assays the method of choice for diagnosing intra-uterine infections in the neonate.

70

ADVANTAGES FOR THE VETERINARIAN

In the medical diagnostic laboratory one is asked to diagnose a considerable number of acute viral infections. This poses problems since for each MACRIA a balanced virus antigen and labelled antibody is needed. On the other hand, only anti-human µFc is required for the solid phase. In contrast, what will be required by the veterinarian is a range of anti-species-specific µFc antisera for coating the solid phase. However, the advantage lies in the next step where a single matched antigen and antibody set will complete the assay for any given virus, irrespective of which species is being investigated.

OTHER USES

Class specific antibody capture assays may be used in a number of ways. The detection of IgM antibody has been described. It is also possible to use an assay with the solid phase coated with anti-γFc to detect IgG antibody (Cohen et al., 1983). This type of assay has also been used to effect in screening for hybridomas secreting antibody to hepatitis B virus antigens (Tedder et al., 1983).

ACKNOWLEDGEMENTS

Figs. 1 - 4 inclusive are reproduced with thanks from the Journal of Medical Virology and Fig. 5 from the Journal of Hygiene. I thank members of this department for helpful discussions.

REFERENCES

Cohen, B.J., Mortimer, P.P. and Pereira, M.S. 1983. Diagnostic assays with monoclonal antibodies for the human serum parovirus-like virus (SPLV). J. Hygiene, 91, 113-130.
Diament, J.A. and Pepys, J. 1978. Immunosorbent separation of IgG and IgM for radioimmunoassay of specific antibodies. In "Affinity Chromatography" (Eds. Hoffman-Ostenkof et al.). (Pergamon Press, Oxford, England). pp. 229-231.
Gerlich, W.H. and Luer, W. 1979. Selective detection of IgM-antibody against core antigen of the hepatitis B virus by modified enzyme immune assay. J. Med. Virol., 4, 227-238.
McFerran, J.B., Dane, D.S., Briggs, E.M., Connor, T. and Nelson, R. 1968. Further investigations on enterovirus-neutralising substance in human and animal sera. J. Path. and Bact., 95, 93-99.
Meurman, O.H., Wiljanen, M.K. and Granfors, K. 1977. Solid-phase radioimmunoassay of rubella IgM antibodies: comparison with sucrose gradient centrifugation test. J. Clin. Microbiol., 5, 257-262.
Morgan-Capner, P., Tedder, R.S. and Mace, J.E. 1983. Rubella-specific IgM reactivity in sera from cases of infectious mononucleosis. J. Hygiene,

90, 407-413.

Pattison, J.R. and Dane, D.S. 1975. The detection of specific IgM antibodies following infection with rubella virus. J. Clin. Pathol., 28, 377-382.

Salacinski, P., Hope, J., McLean, C., Clement-Jones, V., Sykes, J., Price, J. and Lowry. P.J. 1979. A new simple method which allows theoretical incorporation of radioiodine into proteins and peptides without damage. J. Endocrinol., 81, 131-137.

Sutherland, S. and Briggs, J.D. 1983. The detection of antibodies to cytomegalovirus in the sera of renal transplant patients by an IgM capture assay. J. Med. Virol., 11, 147-159.

Tedder, R.S. and Wilson-Croome, R. 1980. Detection by radioimmunoassay of IgM class antibody to hepatitis B core antigen: a comparison of two methods. J. Med. Virol., 6, 235-247.

Tedder, R.S., Yao, J.L. and Anderson, M.J. 1982. The production of monoclonal antibodies to rubella haemagglutinin and their use in antibody-capture assays for rubella-specific IgM. J. Hygiene, 88, 335-350.

Tedder, R.S., Guarascio, P., Yao, J.L., Lord, R.B. and Eddlestone, A.L.W.F. 1983. Production of monoclonal antibodies of hepatitis B surface and core antigens , and use in the detection of viral antigens in liver biopsies. J. Hygiene, 90, 135-142.

DETECTION AND IDENTIFICATION OF PAPILLOMAVIRUSES IN BENIGN
AND MALIGNANT TUMOURS OF CATTLE

M. Saveria Campo

The Beatson Institute for Cancer Research,
Garscube Estate, Bearsden, Glasgow G61 1BD, Scotland

ABSTRACT

Papillomavirus has been isolated from different types of tumours in British cattle. By using restriction enzyme analysis and molecular hybridization six different types of bovine papillomavirus (BPV-1 to 6) have been identified and characterized. Each virus type has been found associated with a particular lesion and their evolutionary relationship has been established. It is concluded that BPVs fall into two subgroups: subgroup A viruses cause fibropapillomas and subgroup B viruses cause true epithelial papillomas. The members of each subgroup are related to one another, but not to the members of the other subgroup. In addition, the presence of viral genomes has been detected by molecular hybridization in tumours non-productive for mature virus progeny.

INTRODUCTION

The application of the new techniques of molecular biology to the field of classical virology has allowed a detailed analysis of papillomaviruses and their role in oncogenesis. Previous studies on papillomaviruses have been seriously hampered by the lack of a tissue culture system suitable for virus replication. Papillomaviruses replicate only in the keratinizing epithelium, and all the various attempts to obtain virus growth in cultured keratinocytes have so far failed, possibly reflecting the defective differentiation of the epithelial cells in vitro. Because of the unavailability of a productive in vitro system, the only source of virus is still the infected animal, making the characterization of the virus and its genome, and the analysis of its functions a rather laborious task. This problem has been partly overcome by the molecular cloning of the viral DNA into bacterial plasmids and its propagation in prokaryotic cells, and by in vitro cell transformation studies.

The presence of virus in productive warts is easily visualized by electron microscopy (see for instance Jarrett et al., 1978a), but obviously it is not possible to distinguish between different virus types on this basis. The use of restriction endonucleases and molecular hybridization in the analysis of the viral genome has shown that the different species of papillomavirus (human, bovine, etc.) are not single entities, as had been thought previously, but are vastly heterogeneous. To-date, twenty four different types of human papillomavirus (HPV) and six different types of bovine papillomavirus (BPV) have been isolated and characterized.

No obvious evidence of the presence of virus is found in certain types of papillomas and papilloma-derived carcinomas (Jarrett et al., 1978b; Jarrett et al., 1980; Orth et al., 1980; Wettestein and Stevens, 1980). No viral particles and no viral antigens can be detected by electron microscopy and immunological techniques respectively, suggesting the lack of virus involvement in the aetiology of these lesions. However, hybridization studies performed on the DNA of these tumours have revealed the presence of viral genomes, thus showing that cells non-permissive for the expression of the virus vegetative functions can nevertheless sustain viral DNA replication and the expression of the transforming functions.

The primary structure of the DNA of both HPV type 1 and BPV type 1 has been determined (Danos et al., 1982; Chen et al., 1982) and the viral genes have been mapped by in vitro cell transformation (Lowy et al., 1980; Campo and Spandidos, 1983; M.S. Campo, unpublished results) and analysis of the viral RNA transcripts (Amtmann and Sauer, 1982; Heilman et al., 1982; Engel et al., 1983; K.T. Smith and M.S. Campo, unpublished results).

These latter aspects of the biology of the papillomaviruses will not be dealt with in this paper, which shall confine itself to the detection, identification and characterization of the bovine papillomaviruses found in benign and malignant tumours of British cattle.

MATERIALS AND METHODS

Tumours

These were obtained either from cattle in a large abattoir or from cattle kept in the Veterinary School, University of Glasgow. They were selected on morphological grounds and removed immediately after slaughter. Specimens were frozen in liquid nitrogen and then stored at -70°C.

Isolation of virions and extraction of viral DNA (Campo et al., 1980; Campo et al., 1981).

Virus isolations was performed on tumours from individual animals; pools were not used. Tumours were cut in small pieces and homogenized in 0.1 M NaCl, 10 mM Tris pH 8.0, 1 mM EDTA (TS) buffer, or, in later cases, in this buffer containing 0.5% NP40 and 0.5% sodium deoxycholate. Cell debris was spun down at 2,000 r.p.m for 5 mins and the supernatant clarified at

10,000 rpm for 15 mins. Virions were either pelleted at 35,000 rpm for 90 mins or banded in a 10-20% sucrose velocity gradient overlying a 1.5 g/cc^3 CsCl pad by centrifuging at 40,000 rpm for 20 mins. In some cases the dialyzed and resuspended virions were centrifuged to equilibrium in CsCl and the virus band at 1.32 g/cc^3 was collected and pelleted at 35,000 rpm for 2.5 h.

The resuspended virions were treated with 50 µg DNase per ml in MES buffer (50 mM MES, 2.5 mM Mg-acetate, pH 7.0) for 2 h at room temperature, made 5 mM EDTA and then lysed with 1% SDS. The viral DNA was extracted twice with phenol-chloroform and precipitated with two volumes of alcohol. After centrifugation the DNA was suspended in 10 mM Tris pH 7.5, 1 mM EDTA (TE).

Extraction of Tumour DNA

DNA was extracted from tumours as described by Chirgwin et al. (1979). Briefly, the tumours were cut in small pieces and homogenized by hand in a mortar in a solution of guanidinium thiocyanate. Cell debris was removed by centrifugation at 10,000 rpm for 10 mins at 10°C. The supernatant was layered on a two-step discontinuous CsCl gradient, with 1.7 g/cc CsCl at the bottom and an equal volume of 1.6 g/cc CsCl at the top. Centrifugation was carried out in a swing-out rotor at 40,000 rpm overnight at 18°C. In these conditions the DNA bands at the interface between the two CsCl solutions. The DNA band was carefully pipetted out, diluted with TE and repeatedly extracted with phenol. After precipitation with ethanol, the final DNA pellet was resuspended in TE.

Restriction enzyme analysis of viral and tumour DNA (Campo et al., 1981).

Restriction endonucleases were purchased from Boehringer, Miles, BRL and Sigma and used according to the specifications of the manufacturers.

The restricted DNA was electrophoresed in slab agarose gels in 36 mM Tris, 30 mM NaH$_2$PO$_4$.2H$_2$O, 1 mM EDTA (E buffer; Loening, 1969); the gels were stained in E buffer containing 0.5 µg/ml ethidium bromide and the DNA fragments were visualized and photographed under short wave uv light.

Blot hybridization (Southern, 1975).

DNA fragments were transferred to nitrocellulose sheets (Millipore or Schleicher and Schull); the blots were preincubated at 60°C for 2 h in

2xSSC-Denhardt solution (SSC = 0.15 M NaCl, 0.015 M Na citrate) (Denhardt, 1966) containing between 50 and 100 µg/ml calf thymus DNA and then hybridized overnight to ^{32}P-labelled nick-translated (Rigby et al., 1977) recombinant DNA probes (see below) in the same mix at 70°. After extensive washing in 1 x SSC at 60°, the blots were exposed to a presensitized X-ray film (Kodax X-Omat) at -70° for varying lengths of time (Laskey and Mills, 1977).

Molecular cloning of BPV DNA (Campo and Coggins, 1982).

The construction of recombinant pAT153-BPV plasmids was carried out under Category I physical containment, in accordance with GMAG guidelines. Escherichia coli HB101 cells harbouring pAT153 (Twigg and Sherratt, 1980) were grown overnight in L broth containing 50 µg/ml ampicillin and 10 µg/ml tetracycline (both from Sigma). The cells were harvested and lysed and pAT153 DNA was extracted and purified according to standard procedures (Wensink et al., 1974). Viral and plasmid DNAs were cleaved with the appropriate single-cut restriction enzyme. Linear plasmid and virus DNA were mixed in (approx.) a 2:1 molar ratio at a plasmid concentration of 60 µg/ml and ligated with T4 DNA ligase (Boehringer Mannheim) at 11°C overnight in 66 mM-EDTA, 10 mM-MgCl$_2$, 100 µg/ml bovine serum albumin, 10 mM-dithiothreitol, 1 mM-ATP. Cleavage and ligation were monitored by electrophoresing an aliquot of the mixtures in a 1% agarose gel in E buffer. The ligated DNAs were used to transfect competent CaCl$_2$-treated E. coli HB101 cells (Wensink et al., 1974). Transformants were selected on L-agar plates containing 50 µg/ml ampicillin, and the colonies were screened for the presence of virus DNA by hybridization (Grunstein and Hogness, 1975; Thayer, 1979) to nick-translated virus DNA. The positive colonies were grown up in 5 ml L broth containing 50 µg/ml ampicillin and 100 µl samples were used for the analysis of plasmid DNA. This was extracted according to the procedure of Birnboim and Doly (1979), and analysed by restriction enzyme cleavage and blot hybridization.

In situ hybridization (Moar and Klein 1978; Moar et al., 1981).

Complementary RNAs (cRNAs) were synthesized using E. coli RNA polymerase and all four ribonucleotide triphosphates labelled with ^{3}H; the final specific activity was 2x10^7 cpm/µg. Cryostat sections were fixed in 3:1 methanol:acetic acid and the DNA denatured with either 0.05N NaOH or brief heat treatment (100°C for 15 seconds). The latter procedure provided better cell morphology. Thereafter, tissues were hybridized with 3 μg/ml ^{3}H-cRNA for 16 h at 60°C in 3xSSC. After hybridization cells were treated with 30 μg/ml pancreatic RNAse at 37°C for 30 mins followed by extensive washing in 2xSSC with a final rinsing in an alcohol series (50-100%) and air-drying. Autoradiography was performed using Ilford K2 emulsion, and autoradiographs were exposed at 4°C for several periods, up to three months. After developing, fixing and washing with distilled water, slides were stained in 6% Giemsa in phosphate buffer pH 6.8.

Occasionally tissues were pre-treated with 100 μg/ml pancreatic RNase before hybridization to test the effect of possible cRNA-RNA binding: this additional procedure, however, did not lead to a reduction in the final autoradiographic signal of positive controls and it was therefore concluded that autoradiographic grains represented DNA-cRNA hybrids.

RESULTS

Molecular heterogeneity and lesion site specificity

Four major types of papillomatosis have been recognised in British cattle (Jarrett et al., 1980): (1) cutaneous fibropapillomatosis; (2) fibropapilloma of the penis; (3) papillomatosis of the udder and teats, and (4) papillomatosis of the upper alimentary tract. Three types of papillomas can be distinguished morphologically and histologically on the skin of the udder; these are frond fibropapilloma, 'rice grain' fibropapilloma, and frond epithelial papilloma (Campo et al., 1981; Jarrett et al., 1984a). Likewise, two different types of tumours are found in the alimentary tract: squamous papilloma and fibropapilloma (Jarrett et al., 1978a; Jarrett et al., 1984b) (Table 1). All of these tumours produce mature infectious virus, with the exception of the fibropapillomas of the alimentary tract. These will be discussed in a later section.

Virus was isolated from each different type of tumour, and viral DNA was extracted and analysed by the use of restriction enzymes. Restriction enzymes are endonucleases that recognize specific nucleotide sequences, and thus cleave the DNA at sites that are specific for each individual DNA type. The products of digestion are discrete fragments that can be visualized either in agarose or acrylamide gels. Identical DNA molecules will be cleaved in the same fashion by any one enzyme, and will display the same fragment pattern.

TABLE 1 Bovine papillomas and their viruses (U.K.). a, compiled from Jarrett et al. (1980 and 1984a); b, from Campo et al. (1981); c, from Jarrett et al. (1984b); d, from Pfister et al. (1979); e, from Campo et al. (1980); f, from Jarrett et al. (1984a).

Subgroup	Type	Tumour	DNA size (Kilobases)	DNA sequence homology with		Immuno cross-reaction[a] with	
				BPV-1	BPV-4	BPV-1	BPV-4
	BPV-1	Penile fibropapilloma[b]	7.9	100%	0%	Complete	None
		Teat frond fibropapilloma[b]					
		Adjacent skin fibropapilloma[b]					
A	BPV-2	Classical skin fibropapilloma[b]	7.9	70%	0%	Complete	None
		Alimentary canal fibropapilloma[c]					
	BPV-5	"Rice Grain" fibropapilloma[b]	7.9	5%	0%	Partial	None
	BPV-3	Skin true papilloma[d]	7.2	0%	50%	n.d.	n.d.
B	BPV-4	Alimentary canal true papilloma[e]	7.3	0%	100%	None	Complete
	BPV-6	Teat true frond papilloma[f]	7.2	0%	20%	None	n.d.

The restriction pattern obtained with the viral DNA from different types of tumours was the same within one tumour type, but not between types. Thus, the DNA of the penile papilloma and of the teat fibropapilloma virus consistently produced the restriction pattern shown in Fig 1A, and the DNA of the skin wart virus, a different pattern, shown in Fig. 1B. Likewise, virion DNA from the other two types of teat tumours and from the alimentary canal papillomas produced unique restriction fragment patterns (not shown). In addition the genomic DNA of the virus from both the alimentary tract and the teat frond papillomas is smaller than the others by approximately 10% (Fig. 2; Table 1), and the same was observed for the genomic DNA of the virus isolated from cutaneous papillomas of Australian cattle (Pfister et al., 1979; Coggins et al., 1983).

The restriction fragments of the viral DNAs produced by several enzymes in double or multiple digestions were ordered in physical genome maps (Fig. 3). The heterogeneity of the maps shows the existence of six distinct virus types, each one associated with a particular tumour, and suggests that the different molecular organization of the several viral genomes may be responsible for the different cytopathological effects observed.

Molecular cloning

The DNA from the several virus types was digested with restriction enzymes which recognize only one site in the viral genome. Thus, BPV-1, BPV-2 and BPV-6 DNA was digested with HindIII, and BPV-4 and BPV-5 DNA with Bam HI (Fig. 3). The bacterial plasmid pAT153 was digested with HindIII or with Bam HI, both of which cleave it only once in the tetracycline-resistance gene, leaving intact the ampicillin-resistance gene. The appropriately cleaved plasmid and viral DNAs were ligated and transfected into bacteria. Ampicillin-resistant, tetracycline-sensitive colonies were selected, and their plasmid analysed. Following digestion of the plasmids with HindIII or with Bam HI, two fragments were obtained: one co-migrating with pAT153 DNA, and a larger one co-migrating with the parental virion DNA (not shown). The DNA fragments were transferred to nitro-cellulose paper and hybridized to the appropriate radioactive viral DNA: only the large fragments co-migrating with virion DNA hybridized strongly (not shown). These results showed that the ampicillin-resistant colonies harboured recombinant pAT153-BPV plasmids (Fig. 4). These recombinants are referred to as pBV followed by the virus type number. Thus pBV1 designates the recombinant plasmid pAT153-BPV-1 DNA.

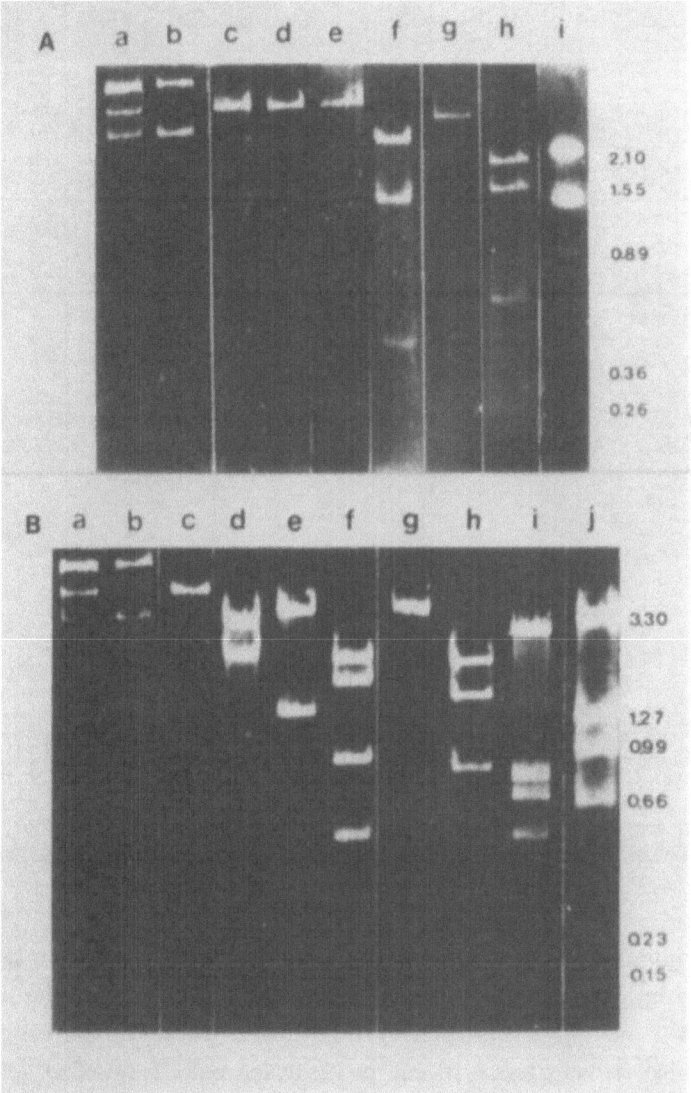

Fig. 1   Restriction enzyme fragments of BPV DNA electrophoresised in a 1.5% agarose gel.
A, virion DNA from teat fibropapilloma, a, no enzyme; b, Sal I; c, EcoRI; d, Hind III; e, Bam HI; f, Bgl II; g, Hind II; h, Hae II; i, Bgl I;
B, virion DNA fron neck fibropapilloma. a, no enzyme; b, EcoRI; c, Hind III; d, Bgl II, e, Bam HI; f, Hind II; g, Hpa I; h, Hae II; i, Bgl I; j, EcoRI- and Hind II- restricted SV40 DNA. The numbers on the right of the photographs are the molecular weights (x10-6) of the standards. Reproduced from Campo et al. (1981)   Virology 113, 323-335, by permission of Academic Press, Inc.

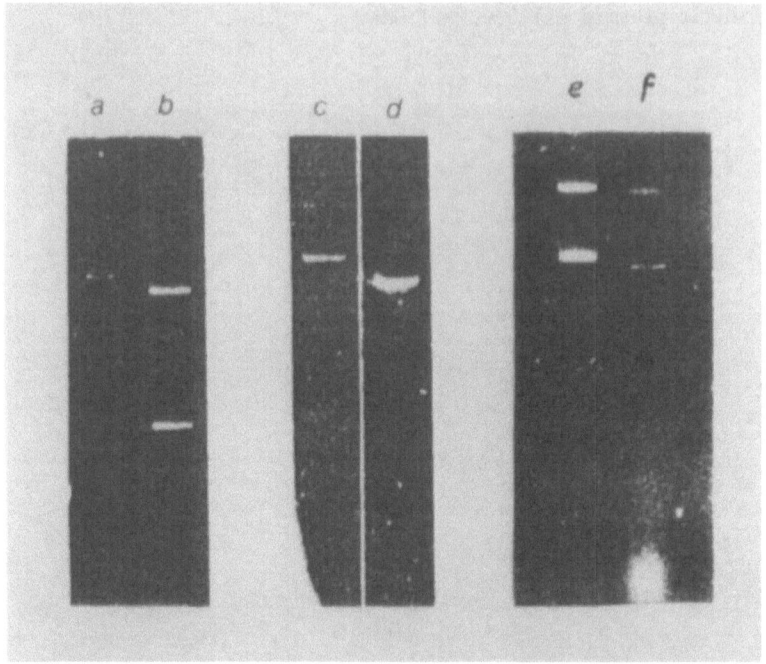

Fig. 2 Comparison between the genomic DNA of BPVs from different
tumours.
a. and e. native virion DNA from neck fibropapillomas; b, native
virion DNA from alimentary tract papillomas; c, Hind III-digested
virion DNA from neck fibropapilloma; d, Bam HI-digested virion DNA
from alimentary tract papillomas; f, native virion DNA from teat
frond papillomas. a-d, reproduced from Campo et al. (1980)
Nature 286, 180-182, by permission of Macmillan Journals Ltd.
e-f, modified from Jarrett et al. (1984a).

The orientation of the viral genomes in the recombinant plasmids was
determined by digestion with several restriction enzymes: the genome of
BPV-1, BPV-5 and BPV-6 was cloned in both orientations, whereas that of
BPV-2 and BPV-4 was cloned in one orientation only (Fig. 4).

    The genome of BPV-3 was cloned using a different strategy. BPV-3 DNA
was digested with EcoRI, which cleaves it only once (Pfister et al., 1979)
and cloned in the EcoRI site of the bacteriophage λ L47 (not shown). The
recombinant phage was digested with EcoRI, and the viral DNA was recloned
in both orientations in the single EcoRI site of pAT153 (Fig. 4).

    The molecular cloning of the BPV genomes achieved two goals; one,
large quantities of viral DNA are now easily available, thus removing the

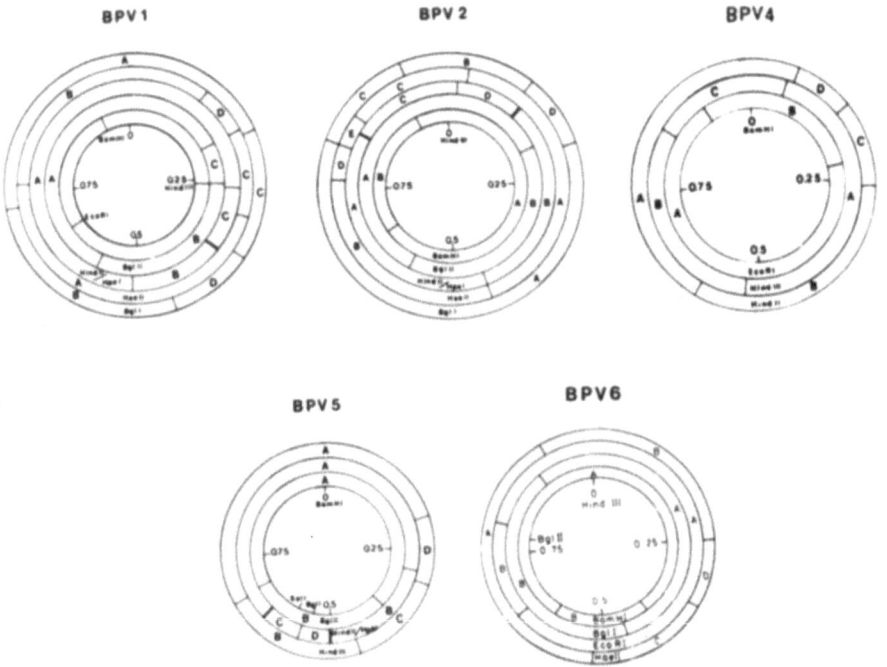

Fig. 3 Restriction enzyme maps of the viral DNA from penile and
teat fibropapillomas (BPV-1); neck fibropapillomas (BPV-2);
alimentary canal squamous papillomas (BPV-4); rice grain fibropapilloma (BPV-5) and teat squamous papillomas (BPV-6). Reproduced
from Campo et al. (1980) Nature 286, 180-182, with permission
from Macmillan Journals Ltd; Campo et al. (1981) Virology 113,
323-335, with permission from Academic Press Inc; and modified from
Jarrett et al. (1984a).
The restriction map of BPV-3 DNA (not shown) was constructed by
Pfister et al. (1979). The different viruses have been designated
type 1 to type 6 according to the accepted nomenclature for
papillomaviruses.

need for infected animals; and two, the viral DNA is free of contaminating
calf sequences, a necessary requirement in hybridization experiments
(see below).

DNA sequence homology between the virus types

The relationship between the several virus types was established by
cross-hybridization experiments between their DNAs. The viral DNAs were
digested with restriction enzymes and the resulting fragments were

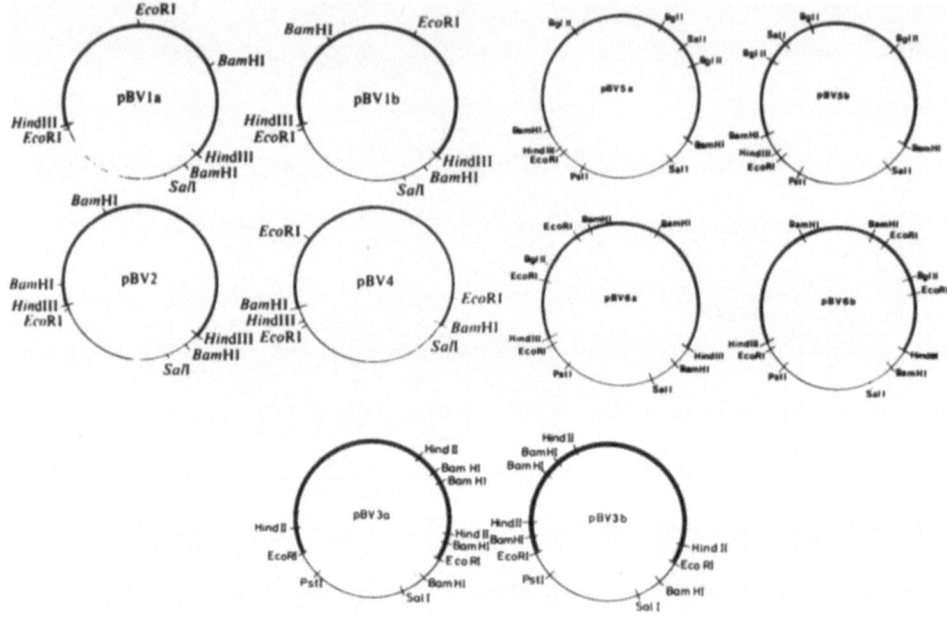

Fig. 4   Restriction maps of the recombinant plasmids. In all cases the thin line represents pAT153 DNA and the thick line represents virus DNA. Only the sites of the relevant restriction sites are shown and the maps are not to scale.
pBV1a and b, pBV2 and pBV4, reproduced from Campo and Coggins (1982); pBV3a and b, modified from Coggins et al. (1983), with permission from the Journal of General Virology; pBV5a and b, M.S. Campo unpublished; pBV6a and b modified from Jarrett et al. (1984a).

transferred to nitrocellulose paper. Each set of fragments was hybridized to the homologous radioactive DNA probe and to each one of the heterologous DNA probes. The results are shown in Fig. 5, and are summarized in Table 1. BPV-1 and BPV-2 DNAs cross-reacted extensively, indicating a high degree of sequence conservation (Fig. 5A), whereas BPV-2 and BPV-5 DNAs did so only partially, showing that these two viruses are only distantly related (Fig. 5B). Neither BPV-1, 2 or 5 DNA cross-hybridized with BPV-3, 4 or 6 DNA (Table 1). However BPV-3 and BPV-4 DNAs showed extensive sequence homology (Fig. 5C), and BPV-6 DNA cross-reacted with both BPV-3 and BPV-4 DNA (Fig. 5D).

These results were confirmed by immuno-crossreaction experiments: BPV-1 and BPV-2 share at least one major antigenic determinant, whereas

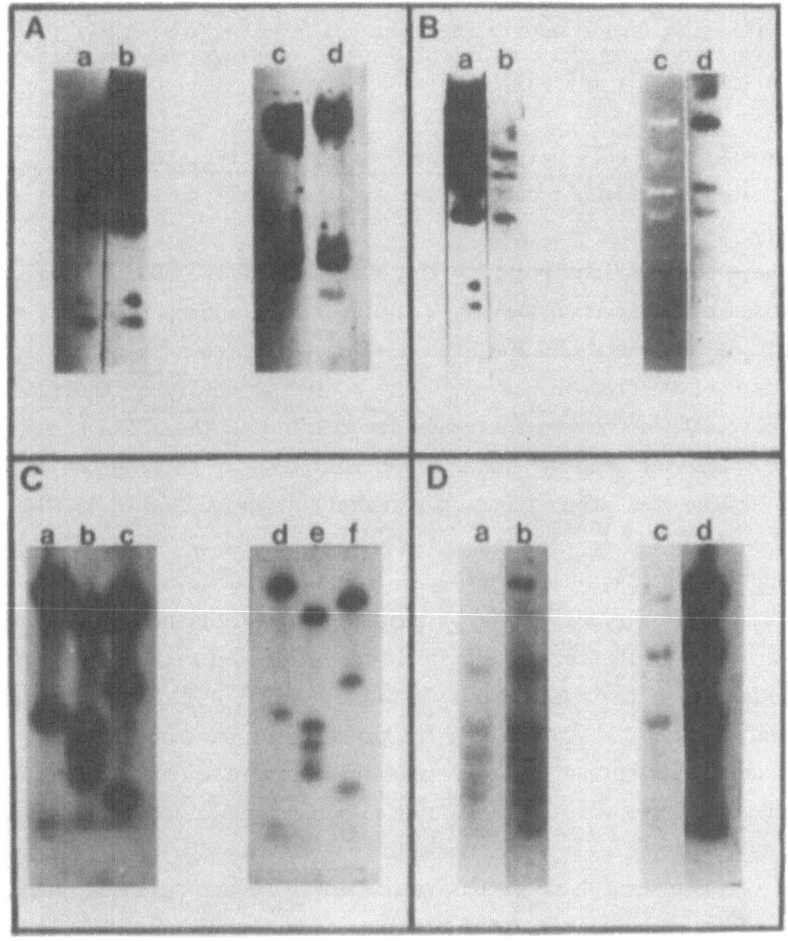

Fig. 5 Sequence homology between viral DNAs.
A, cross-hybridization between BPV-1 and BPV-2 DNAs; a, Hae II
fragments of BPV-2 DNA, hybridized to pBV1 DNA; b, same as a,
hybridized to pBV-2 DNA; c, Hind II fragments of BPV-1 DNA
hybridized to pBV1 DNA; d, as in c, but hybridized to pBV2 DNA.
B, cross-hybridization between BPV-2 and BPV-5 DNAs; a, Hae II
fragments of BPV-2 DNA hybridized to pBV2 DNA and b, to pBV5 DNA;
c, ultraviolet photograph of HindIII fragments of BPV-5 DNA; d,
as in c, hybridized to pBV2 DNA.
C, cross-hybridization between BPV-3 and BPV-4 DNAs; a,b,c, Bam HI,
HindIII and HindII fragments respectively of BPV-3 DNA hybridized
to pBV3 DNA; and d,e,f, to pBV4 DNA.
D, cross-hybridization between BPV-3, BPV-4 and BPV-6 DNAs; a,
HindIII fragments of BPV-3 DNA hybridized to pBV6 DNA, and b, to

pBV3 DNA; c, HindIII fragments of BPV-4 DNA hybridized to pBV6 DNA, and d, to pBV4 DNA.
A and B from Campo et al. (1981) Virology 113, 323-335, with permission from Academic Press Inc; C from Coggins et al. (1983) with permission from the Journal of General Virology and D modified from Jarrett et al. (1984a).

BPV-5 cross-reacts only partially with either of them. Neither BPV-4 or BPV-6 share any antigenic determinant with the first three viruses (Table 1).

These observations point to the existence of two subgroups of BPV. The viruses of subgroup A, BPV-1, 2 and 5, induce fibropapillomas, share antigenic determinants and DNA sequences and have the same genome size. The viruses of subgroup B, BPV-3, 4 and 6, induce wholly epithelial papillomas, have no common antigens, are related in their DNA sequences and have a smaller genome. There is no relationship between the two sub-groups, showing that the viruses have widely diverged (Table 1).

Heteroduplex mapping

The colinearity of the viral genomes was established by hetero-duplex analysis. The recombinant plasmids, digested with Sal I, which cuts asymmetrically in the plasmid but not in the viral DNA (Fig. 4), were denatured, allowed to reanneal in the presence of each one of the other recombinants, and spread for electron microscope examination. pBV1b and pBV2 heteroduplexes were double-stranded along most of their length with the exception of several small non-homology loops (Fig. 6A), showing that the two viral genome share extensive homology and are colinear when aligned at the HindIII site (the cloning site). pBV3b and pBV4 formed more complex heteroduplexes: two equal asymmetrical loops were found at the vector-virus junctions, and loops of variable length were found within the paired viral region (Fig. 6B). Occasionally the two asymmetrical loops were seen hybridizing together (not shown). The loops internal to the viral sequences are regions of non-homology. The two loops at the vector-virus junctions are due to the different cloning site in pBV3 (EcoRI) and pBV4 (Bam HI), showing that the two viral genomes have been permuted. Colinearity is re-established when the EcoRI site of BPV-3 is aligned with one of the two EcoRI sites of BPV-4. pBV6 and pBV4 formed similar hetero-duplexes with non-homology loops within the viral region, and two identical loops at the vector-virus junctions (Fig. 6C), which occasionally

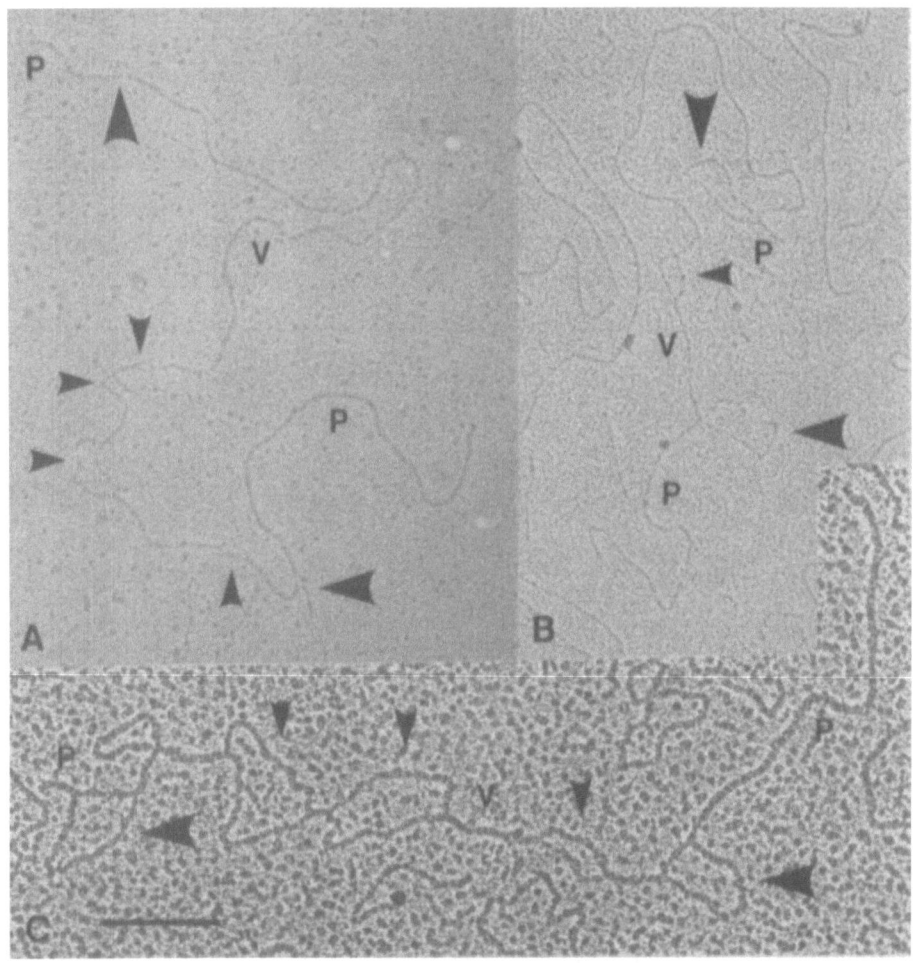

Fig. 6 Heteroduplexes between Sal I-digested pBV1a and pBV2 in
40% formamide (A), pBV3b and pBV4 (B) and pBV4 and pBV6b (C), both
in 35% formamide. P indicates the plasmid regions and V the viral
sequences. The viral genomes hybridize colinearly, except for the
asymmetrical loops (large arrows) at the vector-viral junctions
due to the different restriction sites used for cloning, and for
regions which are denatured (small arrows) due to non-homology
between the two viral genomes. All molecules are shown at the
same magnification and the bar represents 0.25 μm.
B, from Coggins et al. (1983) with permission from the Journal of
General Virology; C, modified from Jarrett et al. (1984a).

hybridized to each other (not shown) indicating that the genomes of BPV-6
and BPV-4 have related sequences and are colinear but are cloned out of
phase. No heteroduplex was ever found between members of the two virus

subgroups in agreement with the results obtained by the blot hybridization technique.

Detection of viral DNA by in situ hybridization

In productive papillomas the presence of viral DNA can be easily demonstrated by in situ hybridization. Large numbers of grains are found in the hyperplastic epithelium, from the stratum spinosum to the stratum corneum (Fig. 7), showing that this is the site of active viral DNA synthesis.

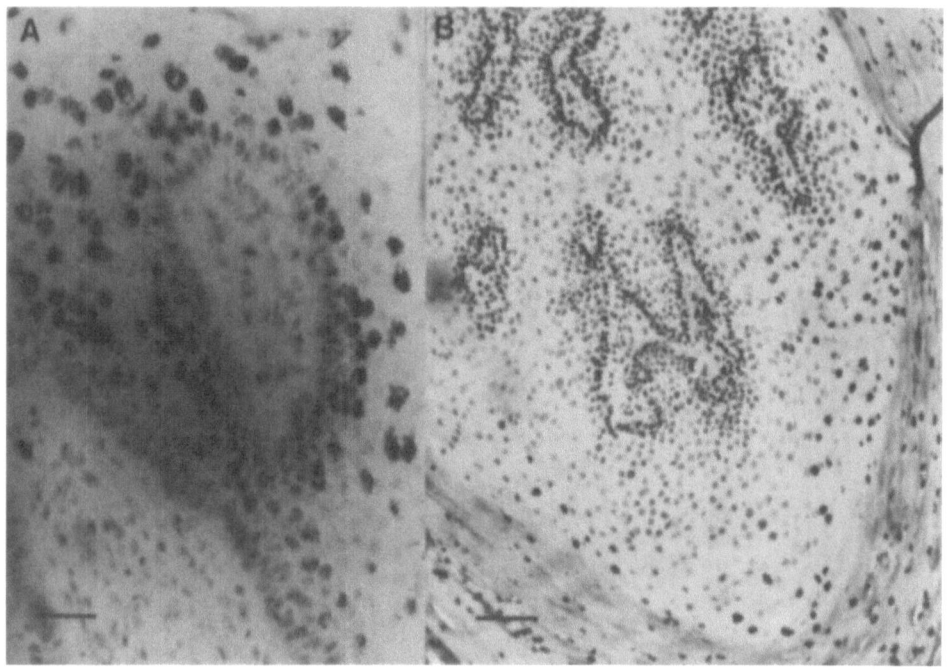

Fig. 7 Detection of viral DNA by in situ hybridization. A, cross section of neck fibropapilloma hybridized to BPV-2 cRNA. The bar represents 3.5 μm. B, cross section of alimentary tract squamous papilloma hybridized to BPV-4 cRNA. The bar represents 7 μm. Photographs, courtesy of Dr. M.H. Moar, Department of Zoology, University of Edinburgh, Edinburgh.

In contrast, no grains are found in the basal cell layer, or in the under-laying derma of fibropapillomas, suggesting that the amount of viral DNA in these cells is too low to be detected by this technique. Thus it would appear that, although transformed, neither the basal cells or the fibro-blasts are permissive for viral DNA replication; judging by the presence of grains, viral DNA synthesis is allowed only when the epithelial cell starts differentiating.

Whereas the viral DNA can be detected throughout the hyperplastic epithelium, the viral capsid antigens are found (by the immunoperoxidase technique, Jarrett et al., unpublished observations) only in the stratum granulosum and in the above layers. Therefore the vegetative functions of the virus are expressed only when the cell starts synthesizing the kera-tohyalin granules, and virus production, from DNA synthesis to virion assembly, is a function of cell differentiation.

Viral DNA in fibropapillomas of the upper alimentary tract

Two types of papillomas are found in the alimentary tract: true squamous papillomas and fibropapillomas. The former are induced by BPV-4 (see above): virus can be seen in the nuclei of the keratinizing layers and can be isolated, and viral antigens and DNA can be detected by the immunoperoxidase and the in situ hybridization technique respectively. In contrast, there is no obvious evidence of virus involvement in the fibropapillomas: no virus and no viral antigens or DNA can be found by the above methods (Jarrett et al., 1984b). These negative results would justify the conclusion for a non-viral aetiology of these tumours, despite their structural similarity to the fibropapillomas induced by BPV-1 and BPV-2. However, when total tumour DNA was digested with restriction enzymes and hybridized to pBV1 or pBV2, the typical banding pattern of BPV-2 DNA was observed in all the specimens examined (Fig. 8), whereas no hybridization to pBV4 was ever detected. These results, while ruling out the involvement of BPV-4, show that, despite the previous contrary evidence, BPV-2 is indeed involved in the production of the alimentary tract fibropapillomas.

It would appear that infection of the alimentary tract by BPV-2 is an abortive process that leads to cell transformation but not to the production of mature infectious viral progeny: whilst permissive for BPV-2 DNA replication, both the epithelium and the underlaying fibroblasts are non permissive for the expression of the viral vegetative functions.

Viral DNA in squamous carcinomas of the upper alimentary tract

In cattle eating the fern bracken, the squamous papillomas of the alimentary tract show a propensity to become the focus for malignant trans-formation into squamous cell carcinomas, thus suggesting a strong co-operative action between a viral agent and environmental factors (Jarrett

88

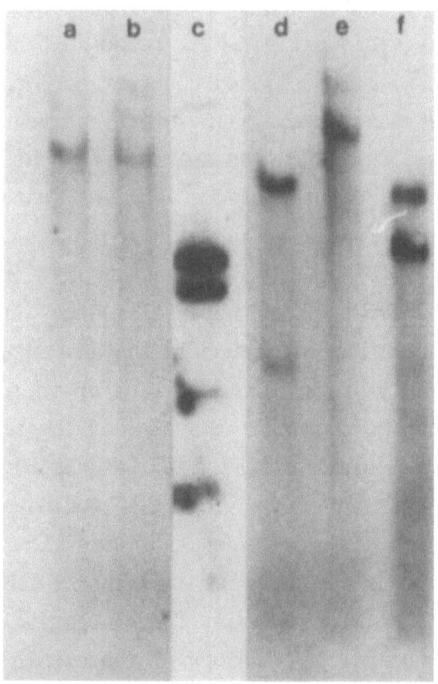

Fig. 8 Detection of viral DNA in alimentary tract fibropapillomas. Tumour DNA was digested with a, no enzyme; b, EcoRI; c, Hind II; d, Bam HI; e, Hind III; f, Bgl II; fractionated in a 1% agarose gel, blotted onto nitrocellulose paper and hybridized to labelled pBV2 DNA. Modified from Jarrett et al. (1984b).

et al., 1978b). These cancers, although derived from virus-induced papillomas, do not produce virions nor do they contain viral antigens (Jarrett et al., 1980). Total DNA from several primary cancers and from metastatic cancers (livers, kidneys, lymphnodes) was analysed for the presence of viral genomic sequences by Southern hybridization. BPV-4 DNA was found in only three cases: two "transforming papillomas", i.e. papillomas with a cancerous centre, and one tongue carcinoma (Fig. 9) where only small amounts of DNA were present. All the other cases proved negative. These results suggest, but do not prove, that the transition from papilloma to carcinoma is accompanied by a progressive reduction of viral expression with ultimate loss of the viral DNA. If this is the case, the transformed state, although presumably induced by the virus, does not require the continuous presence of the virus genetic material. Alternative-ly, the viral genome may still be present in the cancer cells, but below detection levels (less than one copy in ten cells).

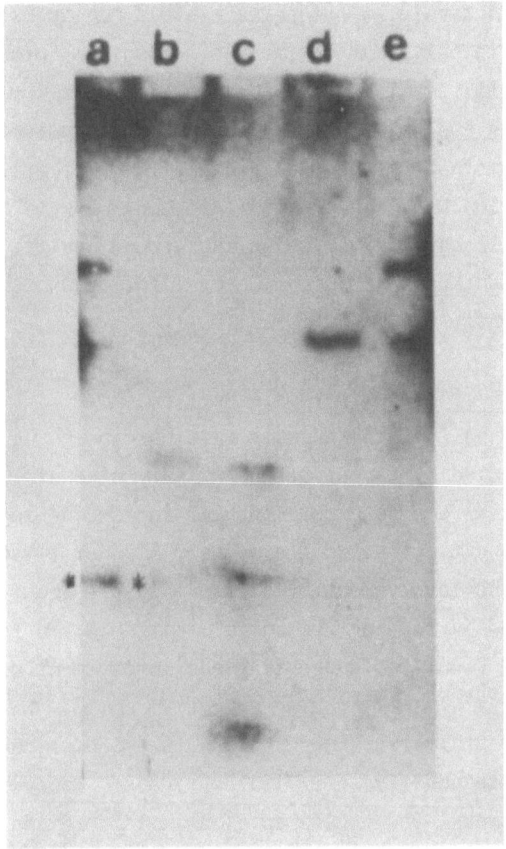

Fig. 9   Detection of viral DNA in alimentary tract squamous carcinoma. Tumour DNA was digested with a, no enzyme; b, EcoRI; c, Hind III; d, Bam HI; e, Bgl II; fractionated in a 1% agarose gel, blotted onto nitrocellulose paper and hybridized to labelled pBV4 DNA.

The sensitivity of the hybridization technique is not the only potential problem. Another problem is cross-hybridization between endogenous plasmid sequences carried by natural bacterial flora and the plasmid moiety of the radioactive recombinant probe. For example, the bands indicated by an asterisk in Fig. 9 detected by the pBV4 probe, were

also seen when tumour DNA was hybridized with labelled pAT153 carrying no
viral sequences. However this problem can be overcome by digesting the
recombinant DNA with the appropriate restriction enzyme (Bam HI in the case
of pBV4), and by separating the viral DNA from the plasmid in a preparative
agarose gel. The viral DNA can then be labelled and used in hybridization
experiments. Alternatively, two duplicate blots can be used, one
hybridized to plasmid only, and one to the recombinant probe. A comparison
of the two blots will reveal which bands are due to the presence of bona
fide viral sequences and which ones to contaminating plasmid. Despite this
inconvenience, recombinant probes are greatly to be preferred to
preparations of virion DNA. These are often contaminated by calf DNA
sequences, which will cause a very high background against which it would
be difficult to detect the hybridization of viral sequences, especially if
present in low amounts.

Viral DNA in cancers of the urinary bladder

Approximately half of the animals with carcinomas of the alimentary
tract are also affected by cancer of the urinary bladder (Jarrett et al.,
1978b). These cancers can be experimentally induced by inoculating
cutaneous papilloma extracts into the urinary bladder (Olson et al., 1959,
1965), suggesting the involvement of a transmissible agent in the genesis
of these tumors; and by feeding the animals with bracken fern (Jarrett
et al., unpublished results), suggesting the involvement of chemical
factors.

Like the alimentary tract carcinomas, the bladder cancers do not
produce virus and are negative for viral antigens. However, when the
tumours from the bracken-fed experimental animals were analysed for the
presence of viral DNA, eight out of nine cases proved to be positive.
All of them harboured multiple copies of BPV-2 DNA (Fig. 10), confirming
Olson's earlier observations and strongly suggesting a synergistic action
between the papillomavirus and the chemical co-carcinogens present in the
bracken.

DISCUSSION

The heterogeneity of bovine papillomaviruses at the molecular and
antigenic level is reflected in the multitude of different tumours of
which they are the causative agents. This diversity presents a potential

problem for the effective management of the disease. Papillomatosis of

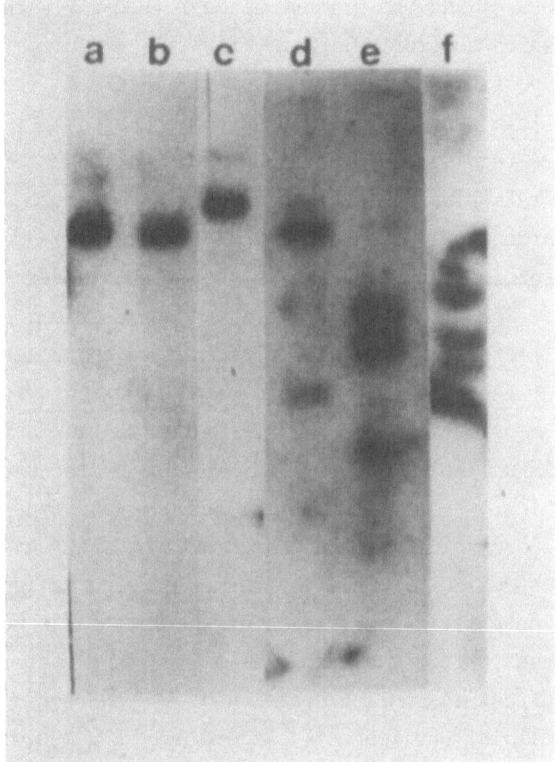

Fig. 10   Detection of viral DNA in urinary bladder cancers.
Tumour DNA was digested with a, no enzyme; b, EcoRI; c, Hind III;
d, Bam HI, e, Hind II; f, Bgl II; fractionated in a 1% agarose gel,
blotted onto nitrocellulose paper and hybridized to labelled
pBV2 DNA.
The BPV-2 DNA present in this cancer is a variant for the Bgl II sites.

the skin of the udder and teats is probably the most common of all the
papilloma lesions, and presents an economic problem as the tumours tend to
persist for long periods and to spread to contiguous areas. The three
types of teat and udder lesions, although superficially similar, are
caused by three very different viruses. For a vaccine to be effective
against, say, the true papillomas, it would have to be raised against
BPV-6, the aetiological agent of the these tumours: vaccines raised
against any of the other viruses would be ineffective as BPV-6 does not
share any antigenic determinants with them. The identification of the
virus is thus the first step towards successful control of the disease.

Papillomaviruses are associated with the malignant cancers of the alimentary tract (BPV-4) and the urinary bladder (BPV-2), although their role in the progression towards malignancy is still obscure. At one end of the spectrum of possible hypotheses for a viral role in the neoplastic process, the virus is a necessary but not sufficient agent: viral infection (papilloma) is a pre-requisite for any subsequent malignant transformation, but this would not take place without the synergistic effect of an environmental co-carcinogen (bracken fern). At the other end of the spectrum, the presence of the viral DNA in, say, the bladder cancers, is only opportunistic. The proliferating malignant epithelium, already triggered by other factors, may provide a permissive environment for viral DNA replication, but the expression of the viral functions would be irrelevant to the neoplastic progression. Circumstantial evidence makes this last hypothesis unlikely, at least in the case of the cancers of the alimentary tract. The two alimentary tract lesions, the true squamous papilloma and the fibropapilloma, are caused by two different viruses, BPV-4 and BPV-2, respectively. Only the former undergo malignant transformation, whereas neoplastic progression of the latter has never been reported. This suggests that the virus is an important factor in carcinogenesis, and that the full expression of its oncogenic potential is linked to its cellular environment. Accordingly BPV-4 would be carcinogenic for the epithelium of the alimentary tract, and BPV-2 for the urinary bladder. Confirmation of the hypothesis should come in the near future.

ACKNOWLEDGEMENTS

This work was carried out with the aid of grants from the Cancer Research Compaign, the Agricultural Research Council and the National Institutes of Health. The author is the recipient of a Cancer Research Campaign Career Development Award.

REFERENCES

Amtmann, E. and Sauer, G. 1982. Bovine papillomavirus transcription: polyadenylated RNA species and assessment of the direction of transcription. J. Virol., 43, 59-66.
Birnboim, H.C. and Doly, J. 1979. A rapid alkaline extraction procedure for screening recombinant plasmid DNA. Nuc. Ac. Res., 7, 1513-1523.
Campo, M.S. and Coggins, L.W. 1982. Molecular cloning of bovine papillomavirus genomes and comparison of their sequence homologies by heteroduplex mapping. J. Gen. Virol., 63, 255-264.

Campo, M.S., Moar, M.H., Jarrett, W.F.H. and Laird, H.M. 1980. A new papillomavirus associated with alimentary cancer in cattle. Nature, London, 286, 180-182.

Campo, M.S., Moar, M.H., Laird, H.M. and Jarrett, W.F.H. 1981. Molecular heterogeneity and lesion site specificity of cutaneous bovine papillomaviruses. Virology, 113, 323-335.

Campo, M.S. and Spandidos, D.A. 1983. Molecularly cloned bovine papillomavirus DNA transforms mouse fibroblasts in vitro. J. Gen. Virol., 64, 549-557.

Chen, E.Y., Howley, P.M., Levinson, A.D. and Seeburg, P.H. 1982. The primary structure and genetic organization of the bovine papilloma-virus type 1 genome. Nature, London, 299, 529-534.

Chirgwin, J.M., Przybyla, A.E., MacDonald, R.J. and Rutter, W.J. 1979. Isolation of biologically active ribonucleic acid from sources enriched in ribonuclease. Biochemistry, 18, 5294-5299.

Coggins, L.W., Hettich, T., Smith, K.T., Slater, A.A., Roe, F.A., Pfister, H. and Campo, M.S. 1983. The genomes of bovine papilloma-viruses types 3 and 4 are colinear. J. Gen. Virol., 64, in press.

Danos, O., Katinka, M. and Yaniv, M. 1982. Human papillomavirus complete DNA sequence: a novel type of genome organization among Papovaviridae. EMBO Journal, 1, 231-236.

Denhardt, K. 1966. A membrane filter technique for the detection of complementary DNA. Biochem. Biophys. Res. Commun., 23, 641-646.

Engel, L.W., Heilman, C.A. and Howley, P.M. 1983. Transcriptional organization of Bovine Papillomavirus Type 1. J. Virol., 47, 516-528.

Grunstein, M. and Hogness, D.S. 1975. Colony hybridization: a method for the isolation of cloned DNAs that contain a specific gene. Proc. Nat. Acad. Sci. USA, 72, 3961-3965.

Heilman, C.A., Law, M.-F., Israel, M.A. and Howley, P.M. 1980. Cloning of human papillomavirus genomic DNAs and analysis of homologous poly-nucleotide sequences. J. Virol., 36, 395-407.

Jarrett, W.F.H., Murphy, J., O'Neill, B.W. and Laird, H.M. 1978a. Virus-induced papillomas of the alimentary tract of cattle. Internat. J. Cancer, 22, 323-328.

Jarrett, W.F.H., McNeil, P.E., Grimshaw, T.R., Selman, I.E. and McIntyre, W.I.M. 1978b. High incidence area of cattle cancer with a possible interaction between an environmental carcinogen and a papillomavirus. Nature, London, 274, 215-217.

Jarrett, W.F.H., McNeil, P.E., Laird, H.M., O'Neil, B.W., Murphy, J., Campo, M.S. and Moar, M.H. 1980. Papillomaviruses in benign and malignant tumours of cattle. In "Viruses in Naturally Occurring Cancers" (Eds. M. Essex, G. Todaro and H. zur Hausen). (New York: Cold Spring Harbor Laboratory). pp. 215-222.

Jarrett, W.F.H., Campo, M.S., O'Neil, B.W., Laird, H.M. and Coggins, L.W. 1984a. A novel bovine papillomavirus (BPV-6) causing true epithelial papillomas of the mammary gland skin: a member of a proposed new BPV subgroup. Virology, submitted.

Jarrett, W.F.H., Campo, M.S., Blaxter, M.L., O'Neil, B.W., Laird, H.M., Moar, M.H. and Sartirana, M.L. 1984b. Alimentary fibropapillomas in cattle. J. Nat. Cancer Inst., submitted.

Laskey, R.A. and Mills, A.D. 1977. Enhanced autoradiographic detection of p^{32} and I^{125} using intensifying screens and hypersensitized film. FEBS Lett., 82, 314-316.

Loening, U.E. 1969. The determination of the molecular weight of ribonucleic acid by polyacrylamide-gel electrophoresis. Biochem. J., 113, 131-138.

94

Lowry, D.R., Dvoretzky, L., Shober, R., Law, M.-F., Engel, L. and
Howley, P.M. 1980. In vitro tumorigenic transformation by a defined
subgenomic fragment of bovine papilloma virus DNA. Nature, London,
287, 72-74.

Moar, M.H. and Klein, G. 1978. Detection of Epstein-Barr virus (EBV) DNA
sequences using in situ hybridization. Biochim. Biophys. Acta.,
519, 49-64.

Moar, M.H., Campo, M.S., Laird, H.M. and Jarrett, W.F.H. 1981. Unintegrated viral DNA sequences in a hamster tumour induced by bovine
papillomavirus. J. Virol., 39, 945-949.

Olson, C., Pamukcu, A.M., Brobst, D.F., Kowalczyk, T., Satter, E.J. and
Price, J.M. 1959. A urinary bladder tumour induced by a bovine
cutaneous papilloma agent. Cancer Res., 19, 779-783.

Olson, C., Pamukcu, A.M. and Brobst, D.F. 1965. Papilloma-like virus from
bovine urinary bladder tumours. Cancer Res., 25, 840-849.

Orth, G., Jabloska, S., Favre, M., Croissant, O., Breitburd, F.,
Obalek, S., Jarzabek-Chorzelska, M. and Rzesa, G. 1980. Epidermo-
dysplasia verruciformis: A model for the role of papilloma-viruses
in human cancer. In "Viruses in Naturally Occurring Cancers" (Eds.
M. Essex, G. Todaro and H. zur Hausen). (New York: Cold Spring
Harbor Laboratory). pp. 259-282.

Pfister, H., Linz, V., Gissmann, L., Huchthausen, B., Hoffmann, D. and zur
Hausen, H. 1979. Partial characterization of a new type of bovine
papillomavirus. Virology, 96, 1-8.

Rigby, P.W.J., Dieckmann, M., Rhodes, C. and Berg, P. 1977. Labelling
deoxyribonucleic acid to high specific activity in vitro by nick
translation with DNA fragments separated by gel electrophoresis.
J. Mol. Biol., 113, 237-251.

Southern, E.M. 1975. Detection of specific sequences among DNA fragments
separated by gel electrophoresis. J. Mol. Biol., 98, 503-517.

Thayer, R.E. 1979. An improved method for detecting foreign DNA in
plasmids of Escherichia coli. Analyt. Biochem., 98, 60-63.

Twigg, A.J. and Sherratt, D. 1980. Trans-complementable copy-number
mutants of plasmid Col El. Nature, London, 283, 216-218.

Wensink, P.C., Finnegan, D.J., Donelson, J.E. and Hogness, D.S. 1974.
A system for mapping DNA sequences in the chromosomes of Drosophila
melanogaster. Cell, 3, 315-325.

Wettstein, F.O. and Stevens, J.G. 1980. Distribution and state of viral
nucleic acid in tumours induced by Shope papillomavirus. In "Viruses
in Naturally Occurring Cancers" (Eds. M. Essex, G. Todaro and
H. zur Hausen). (New York: Cold Spring Habor Laboratory). pp. 301-
307.

DETECTION OF VIRAL NUCLEIC ACIDS IN CELL CULTURES AND IN CLINICAL SPECIMENS BY SPOT HYBRIDIZATION

T. Hyypia[*], P. Stalhandske[**], R. Vainionpaa[*], P. Halonen[*],
U. Pettersson[**].

*Department of Virology, University of Turku
SF-20520 Turku, Finland
**Department of Medical Genetics, University of Uppsala
S-75123 Uppsala, Sweden

ABSTRACT

Nucleic acid hybridization was used for detection of adenovirus DNA directly in clinical specimens and enterovirus RNA in infected cells. DNA in 40 stool specimens, including 18 adenovirus positive and 22 adenovirus negative samples according to a highly sensitive radioimmunoassay (RIA), was spotted onto a nitrocellulose filter and hybridized with radioactively labelled adenovirus type 2 DNA probe. Sixteen specimens positive by RIA and one negative by RIA were positive in the hybridization test. A cloned partial copy of the coxsackie B3 virus genome was used to detect enteroviruses in infected cells. Cells infected with coxsackieviruses A and B, echo and polioviruses gave positive signals in the hybridization assay, whereas cells infected with other viruses did not.

INTRODUCTION

Nucleic acid hybridization techniques have recently been applied successfully to rapid detection of several DNA viruses (Brandsma and Miller, 1980; Stalhandske and Pettersson, 1982; Chow and Merigan, 1983; Virtanen et al., 1983), RNA viruses (Flores et al., 1983) and viroids (Owens and Diener, 1981). In the hybridization test, virus-specific nucleic acids bound onto the solid phase are detected by radioactively labelled DNA probes. We have used the detection of adenoviruses and enteroviruses as model systems to evaluate the possibility of demonstrating viral DNA and RNA in clinical specimens.

MATERIALS AND METHODS

Specimens

Stool specimens used in the adenovirus hybridization test included 18 adenovirus positive and 22 negative samples as determined by radioimmunoassay (RIA) for adenovirus hexon antigen (Halonen et al., 1980). The specimens were diluted 1/10 in PBS, clarified by low speed centrifugation and stored at $-20^{\circ}C$ until assayed.

The specimens for the enterovirus hybridization assay included

LLC-cells infected with coxsackieviruses A9, B2, B3 or B4, echovirus 17 or poliovirus 3. Noninfected LLC-cells, Vero cells infected with herpes simplex virus type 1, adenovirus type 2 or measles virus, and Nebraska calf diarrhoea virus grown in LLC-cells, were included as controls for specificity. Enterovirus isolates from the routine specimen collection were also studied.

The spot hybridization test

The general procedure has been described (Stalhandske and Pettersson, 1982). For the adenovirus hybridization test 200 µl aliquots of stool suspensions were treated with proteinase K (0.1 mg/ml, Merck, West Germany) for 1 h at $37^{o}C$. The suspension was then phenol extracted and the nucleic acids recovered by ethanol precipitation. DNA in the specimen was denatured by boiling at an alkaline pH; specimens were then chilled on ice, neutralized and immobilized on a nitrocellulose filter (Schleicher & Schull, West Germany). The filter was baked at $80^{o}C$ for 2 h and prehybridized for 2 h at $65^{o}C$ in 6xSSC supplemented with 5x Denhardt's solution (Denhardt, 1966) and 50 µg/ml of herring sperm DNA. Purified adenovirus type 2 DNA was labelled with ^{32}P using nick translation (Rigby et al., 1977), denatured and added to the hybridization bag in 6xSSC supplemented with 5x Denhardt's solution and 0.5% SDS; each sample received 100,000 cpm. After hybridization for 16 h at $65^{o}C$ the filters were washed in 2xSSC with 0.5% SDS and the radioactivity bound to the filters detected by autoradiography overnight.

For enterovirus hybridization tests, specimens were treated with proteinase K as above and spotted directly onto the filters. The filter was then baked and prehybridized for 2 h at $42^{o}C$ in 50% formamide, 50 mM Hepes pH 7.4, 3xSSC, 1xDenhardt's solution, 0.1% SDS, 250 µg/ml yeast RNA and 100 µg/ml of herring sperm DNA. A cDNA clone prepared with coxsackie B3 virus RNA as a template was used as the probe (Stalhandske and Pettersson, manuscript in preparation). The cDNA, inserted in E. coli pBR 322 plasmid, was propagated in the HB101 strain of the E. coli. The purified probe was labelled and denatured as above and added to the hybridization bag. After hybridization overnight at $42^{o}C$ the filters were washed and autoradiographed.

RESULTS

Detection of adenovirus DNA in stool specimens

The sensitivity of the test was approximately 100 pg of homologous
DNA. No reaction with nonrelated DNA was observed when DNA from pBR 322
was used as a control.

Forty stool specimens were tested, both by a RIA for the adenovirus
hexon antigen and by nucleic acid hybridization test with an adenovirus
type 2 DNA probe (Fig. 1). Sixteen of the 18 specimens positive according
to RIA were also positive in the nucleic acid hybridization assay and, in
addition, one of the RIA-negative specimens was positive in the hybridization assay (No. 1 in Fig. 1).

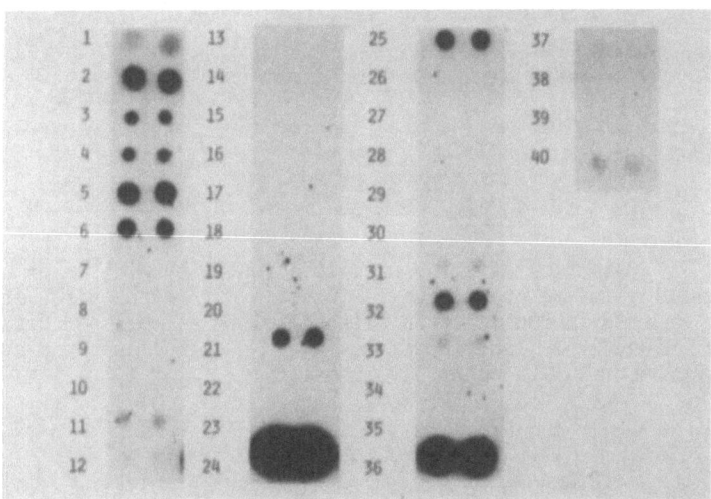

Fig. 1. Detection of adenovirus DNA in 40 stool specimens by spot
hybridization. DNA, isolated from the specimens, was denatured,
spotted in duplicate on a nitrocellulose filter and detected with
an adenovirus 2 DNA probe.

Detection of enterovirus RNA in infected cells

Cells infected with typed virus strains were used to analyse the
specificity of the enterovirus hybridization assay. The probe derived from
coxsackie virus B3 recognised all the enteroviruses tested, although the
signal was rather weak with poliovirus 3 (Fig. 2a). Other viruses did not
react in the assay (Fig. 2b).

In order to evaluate the sensitivity of the hybridization assay for
detection of wild type enteroviruses in clinical specimens, ten coded stool

specimens were inoculated in LLC cells and then tested both by nucleic acid
hybridization and virus isolation. All but one of the eight isolation
positive cell cultures were positive in the spot hybridization test. Moreover, the intensity of the spot was dependent upon the stage of infection
of the cells (data not shown). The isolation negative cell cultures were
both negative in the hybridization test. The eight isolation positive
stool specimens were also tested directly by the spot hybridization assay,
but only one of the samples gave a positive signal.

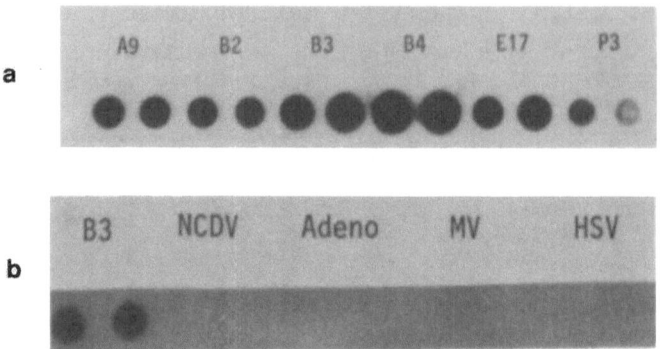

Fig. 2. Detection of viral nucleic acids by hybridization with the
coxsackievirus B3 probe. Cells infected with typed virus strains
were spotted in duplicate on nitrocellulose filters and detected with
the radioactively labelled probe (a). No signal appeared even after
long exposures with control viruses (b).

DISCUSSION

We have evaluated the possibility of detecting viral nucleic acids in
clinical specimens. Adenoviruses in stools were detected with almost the
same sensitivity by direct RIA, which is considered quite sensitive, and
by DNA hybridization techniques. Similar results have also been reported
with sandwich hybridization assay for nasopharyngeal secretion specimens
containing adenoviruses (Virtanen et al., 1983).

In order to detect enteroviruses by nucleic acid hybridization, a coxsackie B3 virus derived probe was used. On the basis of sequence studies
of the cDNA it is known that the insert consists of approximately 4300
base pairs and contains the entire gene for the enterovirus replicase.
This gene is likely to be highly conserved during evolution of the enteroviruses and therefore it is not surprising that our technique was able to
detect all enterovirus strains studied. However, the assay was not sensitive enough to directly detect more than one of eight stool specimens

known to contain enteroviruses. This may be due to the small quantity of virus in the samples or to the presence of ribonuclease activity in the stool specimens. After a single passage in LLC-cells, the hybridization test could easily detect the viral RNA sequences and the results were almost identical obtained by virus isolation. At present, therefore, this assay system can only be used to confirm the enterovirus growth in the cells. However, further refinements may allow virus identification by direct assays.

The nucleic acid hybridization technique is a new and promising addition to the recently developed methods for rapid and direct detection of viral structural components in clinical specimens. Recombinant DNA technology enables the production of probes in almost unlimited quantities. The use of radioactive probes in this assay is still a limitation but new methods for labelling of the probes have recently been developed (Leary et al., 1983) and it is likely that the radioactive probe systems will be replaced in the near future. One of the advantages of the nucleic acid hybridization test is its high specificity and the possibility of producing general reagents to detect whole groups of viruses as well as reagents for subtyping. The hybridization technique may also be very valuable in diagnosis of latent infections, where the production of viral antigens and infectious virions are limited.

ACKNOWLEDGEMENTS

The study was supported by grants from the Swedish Medical Research Council, the Swedish Cancer Society, the Swedish National Board for Technical Development and the Yrjo Jahnsson Foundation.

REFERENCES

Brandsma, J. and Miller, G. 1980. Nucleic acid spot hybridization: rapid quantitative screening of lymphoid cell lines for Epstein-Barr viral DNA. Proc. Natl. Acad. Sci. USA, 77, 6851-6855.
Chou, S. and Merigan, T.C. 1983. Rapid detection and quantitation of human cytomegalovirus in urine through DNA hybridization. N. Engl. J. Med., 308, 921-925.
Denhardt, D.T. 1966. A membrane filter technique for the detection of complementary DNA. Biochem. Biophys. Res. Commun., 23, 641-646.
Flores, J., Boeggeman, E., Purcell, R.H., Sereno, M., Prez, I., White, L., Wyatt, R.G., Chanock, R.M. and Kapikian, A.Z. 1983. A dot hybridization assay for detection of rotavirus. Lancet, i, 555-559.
Halonen, P., Sarkkinen, H., Arstila, P., Hjertsson, E. and Torfason, E. 1980. Four-layer radioimmunoassay for detection of adenovirus in stool. J. Clin. Microbiol., 11, 614-617.

Leary, J.J., Brigati, D.J. and Ward, D.C. 1983. Rapid and sensitive colori-
    metric method for visualising biotinlabelled DNA probes hybridized to
    DNA or RNA immobilised on nitrocellulose: Bio-blots. Proc. Natl. Acad.
    Sci. USA, 80, 4045-4049.
Owens, R.A. and Diener, T.O. 1981. Sensitive and rapid diagnosis of potato
    spindle tuber virioid disease by nucleic acid hybridization. Science
    213, 670-672.
Rigby, P.W.J., Dieckmann, M., Rhodes, C. and Berg, P. 1977. Labelling
    deoxyribonucleic acid to high specific activity by nick translation
    with DNA-polymerase I. J. Mol. Biol., 113, 237-251.
Stalhandske, P. and Pettersson, U. 1982. Identification of DNA viruses by
    membrane filter hybridization. J. Clin. Microbiol., 15, 744-747.
Virtanen, M., Palva, A., Laaksonen, M., Halonen, P., Soderlund, H. and
    Ranki, M. 1983. Novel test for rapid viral diagnosis: Detection of
    adenovirus in nasopharyngeal mucus aspirates by means of nucleic-acid
    sandwich hybridization. Lancet, i, 381-383.

RESTRICTION ENDONUCLEASE ANALYSIS OF AUJESZKY'S DISEASE VIRUS DNA

A.L.J. Gielkens[1], J.T. Van Oirschot[1], F.W. Van Schie[2] and B. Toma[3]

[1]Central Veterinary Institute, Department of Virology,
Houtribweg 39, 8221 RA Lelystad, The Netherlands.
[2]Regional Animal Health Service-Gelderland,
P.O. Box 10, 6880 BD Velp, The Netherlands.
[3]Ecole Nationale Veterinaire d'Alfort,
F-94704 Maisons-Alfort Cedex, France

ABSTRACT

Restriction endonuclease analysis of virus DNA provides a suitable method to differentiate field isolates of Aujeszky's disease virus (ADV). In most cases the differences that have been recognized in cleavage profiles of wild-type strains involved variations in the electrophoretic mobility of certain restriction fragments. Differences with respect to the presence or absence of cleavage sites were less frequently observed. Live-virus vaccine strains of ADV demonstrated unique DNA fragment patterns which were clearly different from one another and from those of wild-type virus isolates.

Restriction endonuclease analysis appeared to be a highly effective tool for (1) the identification of live-virus vaccine and wild-type virus in field cases of AD; (2) the demonstration of structural changes within the virus DNA during attenuation of virulent virus in tissue culture; (3) the study of persistence and spread of ADV within a pig herd and to trace the origin of infection; (4) the identification of the virus(es) excreted after corticosteroid treatment of latently infected pigs.

INTRODUCTION

Aujeszky's disease (pseudorabies) is a clinical disease in pigs manifested by various degrees of nervous disorders, respiratory distress and mortality (Baskerville et al., 1973). The causative agent of AD is a virus classified as a member of the alphaherpesviridae.

Differences in biological properties have been observed among field isolates of ADV (Baskerville et al., 1973). In the past, attempts have been made to find biological markers, such as plaque morphology, heat and trypsin sensitivity to distinguish ADV strains with different virulence properties (Skoda et al., 1964; Bartha et al., 1969). Although some of these in vitro methods allowed differentiation between virulent strains and some vaccine strains, they have not found wide acceptance.

An alternative approach to differentiate herpes virus isolates has been to compare their viral DNAs by restriction endonuclease analysis. This technique was successfully applied in the identification of different isolates of each serotype of herpes simplex virus (Hayward et al., 1975) and proved to be a powerful tool for epidemiological studies (Buchman et al., 1978; Lonsdale et al., 1979).

The genome of ADV has been shown to be a linear double-stranded DNA molecule of approximately 90×10^6 daltons (Rubenstein and Kaplan, 1975). The DNA consists of a short unique sequence (U_S) bracketed by inverted terminal and internal repeat sequences (TR_S and IR_S, respectively) and a long unique sequence (U_L) (Ben-Porat et al., 1979). The short unique region can invert in orientation with respect to the long unique region generating two isomeric forms.

In this report examples are presented of the application of DNA restriction analysis to differentiate field isolates and live-virus vaccines and to resolve questions regarding attenuation, latency and the epizootiology of ADV.

MATERIALS AND METHODS

Isolation of NIA-3 virus DNA

NIA-3 virus was purified from the cell-medium of infected BHK suspension cultures by precipitation with polyethylene glycol and discontinuous sucrose centrifugation. The pelleted virus was resuspended in 50 mM tris-HCl pH 7.8 and 10 mM EDTA and then lysed by the addition of sodium dodecyl sulfate (SDS) to a final concentration of 0.5% and proteinase K (Boehringer) to 100 µg/ml for 2 hrs at 37°C. The extracted virus DNA was purified by 2 cycles of sodium iodide density gradient centrifugation as described by Walboomers and Ter Schegget (1976).

Extraction of infected cell DNA

For the isolation of infected cell DNA, cells were harvested when 70-90% of the monolayer showed a cytopathic effect. Monolayers were washed with a solution containing 10 mM tris-HCl pH 7.4 and 0.15 M NaCl. Cells were harvested by scraping, pelleted by low speed centrifugation and resuspended in 50 mM tris-HCl pH 7.8, 150 mM NaCl and 10 mM EDTA. Proteinase K and SDS were added to final concentrations of 100 µg/ml and 0.5%, respectively. The lysates were incubated at 37°C for 2 hrs and then extracted twice with a mixture of phenol:m.cresol:8-hydroxyquinoline (100:14:0.1) saturated with 50 mM tris-HCl pH 7.8 and twice with chloroform:isoamyl alcohol (24:1). The nucleic acids were ethanol-precipitated and dissolved in 10 mM tris-HCl pH 7.8 and 1 mM EDTA. This DNA preparation was then incubated with 20 µg/ml of pancreatic ribonuclease (Boehringer) for 1 hr at room temperature, followed by incubation with 100 µg/ml of proteinase K for 1 hr at 37°C. The solution was extracted twice with chloroform-isoamyl alcohol and the DNA precipitated with ethanol. The precipitate was dissolved in 10 mM tris-HCl pH 7.4 and 1 mM EDTA.

Restriction endonuclease digestion and electrophoresis of DNA

Restriction endonucleases were purchased from Bethesda Research Laboratories. All digestions were performed at 37°C for 2 hrs in the buffer system recommended by the manufacturer. The reactions were stopped by the addition of 1/5 volume of 50 mM EDTA (pH 7.4), 2.5% SDS, 50% glycerol and 0.125% bromophenol blue, and heating of the samples to 65°C for 10 mins.

DNA restriction endonuclease fragments were electrophoresed at 1V/cm for 40 hrs on 0.6% horizontal agarose gels in 40 mM tris-acetate pH 7.9, 5 mM sodium acetate, 1 mM EDTA and 0.5 µg/ml of ethidium bromide (Berns et al., 1980).

Filter hybridization

Transfer of DNA from agarose gels to nitrocellulose filters and hybridization was carried out essentially as described (Southern, 1975; Quint et al., 1981). The DNA in the agarose gels was denatured by soaking the gel in 0.5 M NaOH, 1.5 M NaCl for 45 mins, then neutralized with 0.5 M tris-HCl pH 6.0, 1.5 M NaCl for an additional 45 mins and transferred to BA-85 nitrocellulose filter paper (Schleicher and Schull) overnight with 10x SSC (1x SSC is 0.15 M NaCl and 5 mM sodium citrate). After blotting, filters were rinsed in 2x SSC, dried at room temperature and baked under vacuum for 4 hrs at 80°C.

The filters were preincubated for 4 hrs at 42°C in 50% formamide, 5x SSC,0.25 mg/ml of denatured salmon sperm DNA, 50 mM sodium phosphate pH 7.0 and Denhardt's solution (Denhardt, 1966). Hybridization was carried out in a solution containing 50% formamide, 5x SSC, 1 mM EDTA, 0.1 mg/ml of denatured salmon sperm DNA, 20 mM sodium phosphate pH 7.0, Denhardt's solution and 0.2×10^6 to 0.5×10^6 cpm/ml of purified NIA-3 virus DNA labelled with ^{32}P by nick translation (Rigby et al., 1977; Berns et al., 1980). The DNA probe was heat denatured in 70% formamide at 100°C for 10 mins. Hybridization was performed for 16 hrs at 42°C.

After hybridization, the filters were washed three times at 42°C in hybridization solution and twice in 0.1 x SSC containing 0.1% SDS at 42°C.

The nitrocellulose filters were allowed to dry and exposed at -70°C to X-ray film with Dupont Cronex Lightning-Plus intensifying screens.

RESULTS AND DISCUSSION
Procedures for restriction endonuclease analysis

A number of procedures are available to prepare restriction endonuclease fingerprints of ADV DNA. We will briefly discuss three methods of which the first two are most frequently applied for differentiation of virus strains.

In the first method the analysis is carried out using unlabelled DNA. For the preparation of DNA, virions are pelleted from the cell-free culture medium of infected cell cultures by ultracentrifugation. After suspension of virus pellets in a tris-EDTA buffer, virus DNA is extracted by SDS and phenol (Ludwig et al., 1982).

In the second method, virus DNA is labelled in vivo with ^{32}P - orthophosphate. The medium, containing virus released from the cells, and the cytoplasmic extract of NP-40 lysed cells are combined and virus is pelleted by centrifugation. The ^{32}P-labelled virus DNA is extracted by SDS and phenol (Preston et al., 1978).

Both procedures yield viral DNA in sufficient purity for studies aimed to differentiate ADV viral genomes. After restriction endonuclease digestion DNA fragments are separated according to size by electrophoresis through an agarose gel. The position of DNA fragments within the gel can be determined by staining of the gel with ethidium bromide (first technique) or autoradiography (second technique).

In the third procedure total infected cell DNA is cleaved by restriction enzymes. Cells are collected when the virus infected monolayer shows a maximum cytopathic effect. After extraction with SDS and phenol, the total infected cell DNA is digested with a restriction endonuclease and DNA fragments are separated by electrophoresis through an agarose gel. Then the DNA fragments are denatured, transferred to a nitrocellulose filter employing the technique described by Southern (1975) and immobilized. The DNA attached to the filter is then hybridized to ^{32}P -labelled viral DNA and the position of the DNA fragments complementary to the probe is visualized by autoradiography.

The first method, using unlabelled viral DNA, is especially of interest for routine laboratories lacking the facilities to work with radio-isotopes.

This method allows differentiation of wild-type virus and live-virus vaccine, but is only to a limited degree suited for interpretation of changes observed in the DNA fragment patterns.

A very convenient method of differentiating viral genomes is by use of ^{32}P-labelled virus DNA. A minimum amount of DNA is loaded into the slots of the gel by which trailing and smearing of bands is prevented and excellent resolution is obtained. Usually, infection and labelling of only one confluent monolayer in a 25 cm^2 plastic flask is required for the analysis of a particular strain.

An alternative strategy is to identify viral DNA fragments in digests of total cell DNA by blot hybridization.

It is obvious that the blot hybridization procedure will be generally the most laborious one. Compared to the second technique, however, this method has the clear advantage of avoiding the use of large quantities of ^{32}P-orthophosphate to label viral DNAs. In addition to demonstrate that fragments showing size variation from one isolate to another contain corresponding sequences and to identify new fragments resulting from additional cleavage, blots can be reused for probing with isolated or cloned DNA fragments.

Generally, one tissue culture passage of a primary isolate, from for example swabs, suffices to analyze its genome by the latter technique. In this way, the chance of introducing genome alterations is reduced to a minimum.

Differentiation of ADV wild-type virus and live-virus vaccine

The results of studies aimed to differentiate ADV strains and modified live-virus vaccine strains of ADV have demonstrated that restriction endonuclease analysis of viral DNA provides a method for unambiguous identification of ADV isolates (Gielkens and Berns, 1982; Ludwig et al., 1982; Geck et al., 1982; Gielkens et al., in preparation).

For our studies the restriction endonuclease BamHI was chosen because firstly it generates a distinctive pattern of 14 major fragments varying in size from approximately 1 to 30 kb and secondly the positions of the restriction sites in the genome are known (Rixon and Ben-Porat, 1979).

The differences after BamHI cleavage among various wild-type isolates of ADV involved the gain of an additional restriction site in DNA fragments 1, 2 and 3 and obvious changes in the migration of fragments 5, 10, 12, 13 and probably 8'.

All live-virus vaccine strains presently examined, including the strains Ercegovac, MK-25 (Tatarov, 1968), Ay-vak, Duvaxyn, the latter is based on the K-61 strain of Bartha (1961) and Delsuvac, based on strain BUK TK/650-A (Skoda et al., 1964), demonstrated unique fragment profiles that enabled their differentiation from virulent strains (Gielkens et al., in preparation). Compared to the cleavage profile of the virulent strain NIA-3, vaccine strains showed considerable changes involving loss of fragments and/or acquisition of new fragments.

In the course of this study we obtained several isolates derived from pigs showing clinical symptoms of AD shortly after vaccination. In only two of these cases the isolates were identified as vaccine virus. Both isolates were derived from brain tissue and collected several years ago. Since they were plaque purified the simultaneous presence of wild-type virus could not be excluded. Therefore there is no firm evidence that these live-virus vaccines were causing the disease. All isolates derived from more recent cases showed a wild-type virus cleavage pattern.

Analysis of genome alterations introduced during attenuation

A thermosensitive strain (Alfort 26) of ADV was obtained by Toma (1979) after serial passage at low temperature and at terminal dilutions of a virulent field isolate (Alfort 37). During serial passage the culture temperature was stepwise decreased to $26^\circ C$, which was reached at passage level 136. The Alfort 26 strain (passage level 220) is avirulent in sheep and pigs but remains pathogenic in laboratory animals (Toma et al., 1979).

To examine the effect on virus DNA of cell passage at low temperatures, DNA from isolates at passage levels 60, 70, 220, 385 and 500 was cleaved with BamHI. When compared to Alfort 37, no changes were observed in the number of restriction fragments at the different passage levels (Fig. 1). However, both the BamHI digest and the BamHI/KpnI double digest showed that the electrophoretic mobility of some fragment bands gradually increased with increasing passage level. This applied to fragments 10 and 12, which span the junctions between the unique short region (U_S) and the internal (IR_S) and terminal (TR_S) inverted repetitions, respectively, and fragment 5' which is located in the terminal part of the long unique sequence (U_L). Compared to the parent strain, virus at passage level 500 showed deletions of about 100-200 bp in fragments 10 and 12, and of about 200-400 bp in fragment 5'. The greatest change in the size of fragments 10 and 12 occurred during the first 220 passages. It is obvious that additional studies are necessary to examine whether these deletions are of any biological significance.

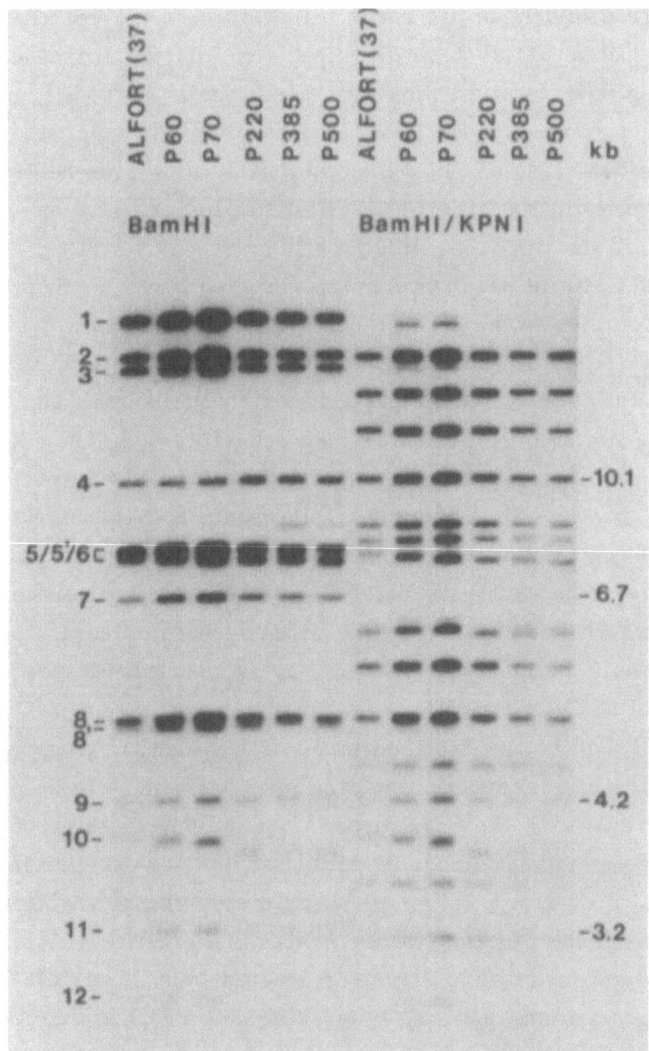

Fig. 1   Autoradiograph of the BamHI and BamHI/KpnI restriction endonuclease digests of DNA from different passage levels of the Alfort (37) strain.

Analysis of epidemiologically related ADV-isolates

Buchman et al. (1978) have reported the application of restriction endonuclease fingerprinting to study temporal clusters of HSV-1 infections.

By this technique they could readily discriminate between isolates belonging to the temporal clusters of hospital infections and unrelated strains.

This type of analysis may also be a valuable asset to study persistence and spread of ADV in pig herds. Therefore, a pig fattening farm where clinical AD had regularly been diagnosed was followed for an 8 month period. The fattening unit received pigs from one breeding farm. During the period of examination oropharyngeal (OP) fluid samples were collected from pigs showing clinical signs of AD, but occasionally also from healthy pigs. Virus was demonstrated in 9 out of 64 OP-fluid samples examined and in the tissues of one of the pigs that died.

The first severe signs of AD were observed among a group of pigs (group I) about 6-7 weeks after the start of the fattening period. Virus was isolated from 6 OP-fluid samples and from tissue specimens of one pig that died. The BamHI cleavage patterns of these isolates showed no differences in the number or location of cleavage sites (Fig. 2). With one exception (sw-1), the patterns also revealed no significant variation in the mobility of corresponding fragments. The small mobility shift observed in isolate sw-1 occurred in the highly variable DNA fragments 10 and 12. We assume, therefore, that these first 7 isolates were representatives of one genotype of ADV. To facilitate the discussion the cleavage patterns of the brain/tonsil isolate and of sw-2, -3, -4, -7 and -10 were designated as type A and of sw-1 as type A'.

Two weeks after the first outbreak of AD, another group (group II) of fattening pigs was introduced into the same building. These pigs were in indirect contact with the first group. Approximately three weeks after the start of the fattening period, OP-fluid samples were collected from 4 pigs of group II. Although no signs of AD were observed at that time, the OP-fluid sample of one pig (sw-15) was positive for virus isolation. The DNA fingerprint pattern of this virus, designated type B, was clearly different from the first isolates. Three days later group II was vaccinated with the live-virus vaccine Delsuvac, which is based on the BUK TK/650-A strain. Shortly afterwards, many pigs showed signs indicative of AD. Eleven days after vaccination group II was sampled again. The virus isolated from one OP-fluid sample (sw-19) showed a type A' pattern, which is clearly different from that of Delsuvac. Afterwards virus was isolated on only one occasion on this farm and again from group II. As with the preceding isolate this virus (sw-26) showed a type A' cleavage profile. Although the data

obtained are still limited, they confirm the usefulness of this type of
analysis for identification and tracing of ADV strains within a herd.

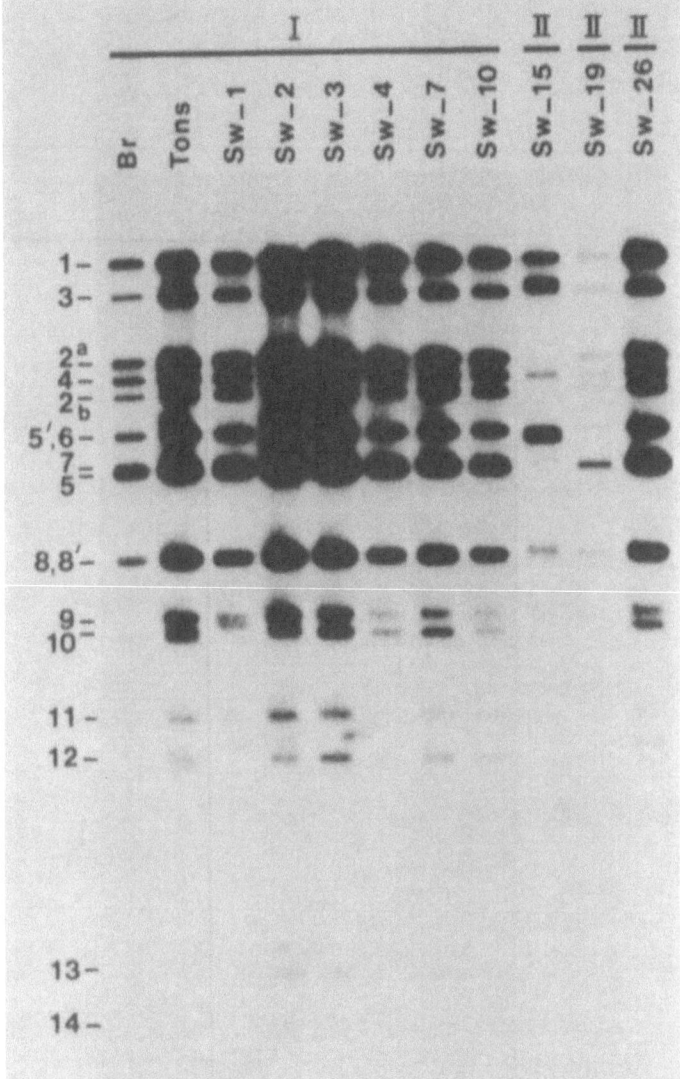

Fig. 2   Autoradiographs of the cleavage profiles of ADV DNA's prepared from isolates collected during a 8 month period on a pig fattening farm.   The DNA's were digested with BamHI.   A detailed description
of these isolates is given in the text.

Analysis of genomes of reactivated ADV

The DNA restriction endonuclease technique has also proved its usefulness in studies aimed to investigate the establishment and reactivation of

110

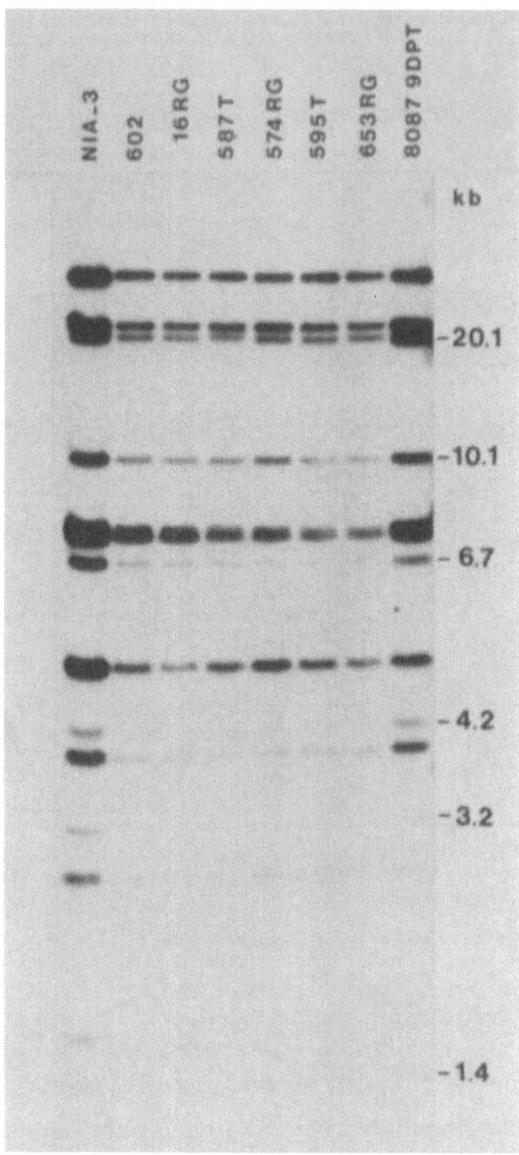

Fig. 3 The DNA cleavage profiles of isolates of the ADV strain NIA-3 from different pigs. DNA preparations were digested with BamHI. At the time of the initial infection with NIA-3, pigs had high, low or no maternal antibody titres. The isolates shown were derived from a brain specimen of pig 602 shortly after infection, from explant cultures of tonsils (587T, 595T) and trigeminal ganglia (16RG, 574RG, 653RG) collected after corticosteroid administration, 4-5 months after infection, and from an OP-fluid sample of pig 8087 nine days after corticosteroid treatment.

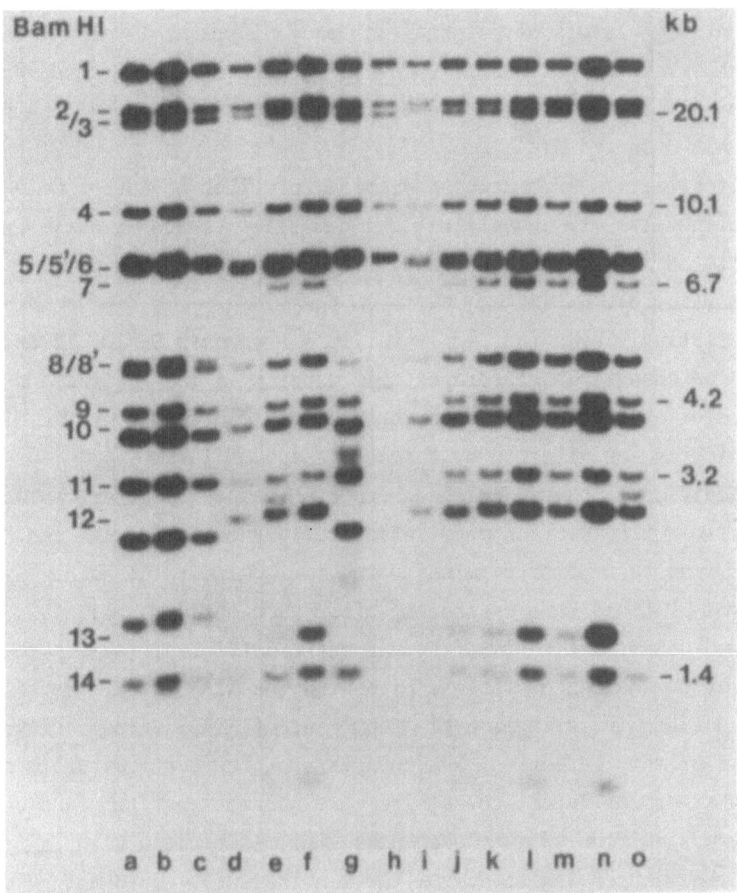

Fig. 4   Autoradiograph of BamHI restriction endonuclease digests of DNA of ADV isolated from OP-fluid samples. Isolates from pigs 8045 and 8056 after intranasal vaccination with Bartha's K strain (lane b, 1DPV; c, 4DPV and g, 3DPV; h, 4DPV, respectively), after challenge exposure with the virulent NIA-3 strain (lane d, 2DPC and i, 3DPC; j, 4DPC, respectively), and after corticosteroid treatment (lane e, 6DPT and k, 9DPT, respectively). Isolates from pigs 8130 (lane f, 13DPT) and 8113 (lanes l, 11DPT and m, 12DPT), which were placed in-contact with pigs 8045 and 8056 respectively, at the time of cortico-steroid treatment. A plaque-purified Bartha virus isolate (lane a), the NIA-3 parental stock (lane n) and a NIA-3 isolate from an oral swab 2 days after primary infection (lane o). Different autoradio-graphic exposures of the blot are combined to show faint DNA fragments.

112

latent ADV in pigs (Van Oirschot and Gielkens, in press). These studies showed that high levels of maternal antibody, intranasal vaccination with Bartha's K strain or parenteral vaccination with an inactivated vaccine failed to uniformly prevent the establishment of latency of the highly virulent NIA-3 strain of ADV.

The restriction endonuclease cleavage profiles of latent NIA-3, reactivated in vitro from ganglionic and tonsillar tissue of different pigs, appeared to be indistinguishable from virus isolated shortly after primary infection (Fig. 3).

Interestingly even the highly variable fragments 5, 10, 12 and 13 demonstrated no changes in electrophoretic mobility. The restriction endonuclease cleavage pattern is apparently a stable property of the NIA-3 strain which is not affected by animal passage or latency.

In addition we have examined whether ADV excreted after challenge and corticosteroid treatment of pigs intranasally vaccinated with the K-strain of Bartha, was vaccine or virulent virus, or a mixture of both. Virus isolated from OP-fluid samples shortly after vaccination of pigs 8045 and 8056 showed a Bartha-like DNA fragment pattern (Fig. 4). Virus recovered a few days after challenge of these pigs with the NIA-3 strain revealed a cleavage pattern indistinguishable from that of NIA-3 virus isolated shortly after a primary infection. At the start of the corticosteroid treatment, ten weeks after challenge, these pigs were housed separately and one sentinel pig was introduced into each pen. The reactivated viruses from both pigs and the viruses isolated from the sentinel pigs could not be distinguished from NIA-3. There was no evidence of simultaneous shedding of vaccine and challenge virus.

ACKNOWLEDGEMENTS

We are very grateful to Dr. D. Todd for critical reading of the manuscript, to Mr. J. Briaire and Miss M. Veldhuis for excellent technical assistance and to Mr. J. Dekker for the photographic material.

REFERENCES

Bartha, A. 1961. Experimental reduction of virulence of Aujeszky's disease virus. Magy. Allatorv. Lap., 16, 42-45.
Bartha, A., Elak, S. and Benyeda, J. 1969. Trypsin- and heat-resistance of some strains of the herpesvirus group. Acta Vet. Hung., 19, 97-99.
Baskerville, A., McFerran, J.B. and Dow, C. 1973. Aujeszky's disease in pigs. Vet. Bull., 43, 465-480.

Ben-Porat, T., Rixon, R.J. and Blankenship, M.L. 1979. Analysis of the structure of the genome of pseudorabies virus. Virology, 95, 285-294.

Berns, A.J.M., Lai, M.H.T., Bosselman, R.A., McKennett, M.A., Bacheler, L.T., Fan, H., Robanus Maandag, E.C., Van der Putten, H. and Verma, I.M. 1980. Molecular cloning of unintegrated and a portion of integrated Maloney murine leukemia viral DNA in bacteriophage lambda. J. Virol., 36, 254-263.

Buchman, T.G., Roizman, B., Adams, G. and Stover, B.H. 1978. Restriction endonuclease fingerprinting of herpes simplex virus DNA: a novel epidemiological tool applied to a nosocomial outbreak. J. Inf. Dis., 138, 488-498.

Denhardt, D.T. 1966. A membrane filter technique for the detection of complementary DNA. Biochem. Biophys. Res. Commun., 23, 641-646.

Geck, P., Nagy, E. and Lomniczi, B. 1982. Differentiation between Aujeszky's disease virus strains of different virulence by restriction enzyme analysis of the DNA. Magy. Allatorv. Lap., 37, 651-656.

Gielkens, A.L.J. and Berns, A.J.M. 1982. Differentiation of Aujeszky's disease virus strains by restriction endonuclease analysis of the viral DNA's. In "Current Topics in Veterinary Medicine and Animal Science" (Ed. G. Wittmann and S.A. Hall). (The Hague, Martinus Nijhoff). Vol. 17, pp. 3-13.

Hayward, G.S., Frenkel, H. and Roizman, B. 1975. Anatomy of herpes simplex DNA: strain differences and heterogeneity in the locations of restriction endonuclease cleavage sites. Proc. Nat. Acad. Sci. USA, 72, 1768-1772,

Lonsdale, D.M., Brown, S.M., Subak-Sharpe,J.H., Warren, K.G. and Koprowski, H. 1979. The polypeptide and the DNA restriction enzyme profiles of spontaneous isolates of herpes simplex virus type 1 from explants of human trigeminal, superior cervical and vagus ganglia. J. Gen. Virol., 43, 151-171.

Ludwig, H., Heppner, B. and Herrmann, S. 1982. The genomes of different field isolates of Aujeszky's disease. In "Current Topics in Veterinary Medicine and Animal Science" (Ed. G. Wittmann and S.A. Hall). (The Hague, Martinus Nijhoff). Vol. 17, pp.15-20.

Van Oirschot, J.T. and Gielkens, A.L.J. In vivo and in vitro reactivation of latent pseudorabies virus in pigs born to vaccinated sows. Am. J. Vet. Res., in press.

Van Oirschot, J.T. and Gielkens, A.L.J. Intranasal vaccination of pigs against pseudorabies. 2. Absence of vaccine virus latency and failure to prevent latency of virulent virus. Am. J. Vet. Res., in press.

Preston, V.G., Davison, A.J., Marsden, H.S., Timbury, M.C., Subak-Sharpe, J.H. and Wilkie, N.M. 1978. Recombinants between herpes simplex virus type 1 and 2: analysis of genome structures and expression of immediate-early polypeptides. J. Virol., 28, 499-517.

Quint, W., Quax, W., Van der Putten, H. and Berns, A. 1981. Characterization of AKR murine leukemia virus sequences in AKR mouse substrains and structure of integrated recombinant genomes in tumor tissues. J. Virol., 39, 1-10.

Ribgy, P.W.J., Dieckmann, M., Rhodes, C. and Berg, P. 1977. Labelling deoxyribonucleic acid to high specific activity in vitro by nick-translation with DNA polymerase I. J. Mol. Biol., 113, 237-251.

Rixon, F.J. and Ben-Porat, T. 1979. Structural evolution of the DNA of pseudorabies-defective viral particles. Virology, 97, 151-163.

Rubenstein, A.S. and Kaplan, A.S. 1975. Electron microscopic studies of the DNA of defective and standard pseudorabies virions. Virology, 66, 385-392.

Skoda, R., Brauner, I., Sadecky, E. and Mayer, V. 1964. Immunisation against Aujeszky's disease with live vaccine. I. Attenuation of virus and some properties of attenuated strains. Acta Virol., Praque, $\underline{8}$, 1-9.

Southern, W.M. 1975. Detection of specific sequences among DNA fragments separated by gel electrophoresis. J. Mol. Biol., $\underline{98}$, 503-517.

Tatarov, G. 1968. Apathogener mutant des Aujeszky-virus, induziert von 5-Jodo-2-Deoxyuridin (JUDR). Zentbl. Vet. Med., $\underline{15B}$, 847-853.

Toma, B. 1979. Obtention et caractérisation d'une souche thermosensible de virus de la maladie d'Aujeszky (Souche Alfort 26). Rec. Méd. Vét., $\underline{155}$, 131-137.

Toma, B., Brun, A., Chappuis, G. and Terre, J. 1979. Propriétés biologiques d'une souche thermosensible (Alfort 26) de virus de la maladie d'Aujeszky. Rec. Méd. Vét., $\underline{155}$, 245-252.

Walboomers, J.M.M. and Ter Schegget, J. 1976. A new method for the isolation of herpes simplex virus type 2 DNA. Virology, $\underline{74}$, 256-258.

PROTEIN BLOTTING: THE BASIC METHOD AND ITS ROLE IN VIRAL DIAGNOSIS

A.J. Herring and J.M. Sharp

Moredun Research Institute, 408 Gilmerton Road,
Edinburgh EH17 7JH, Scotland.

ABSTRACT

Protein blotting involves the transfer of a complex mixture of antigens which have been resolved in a polyacrylamide gel on to a nitrocellulose membrane where the various antigenic components are accessible to
analysis with antibody. The technique can be used to detect viral antigens or to dissect the humoural response to pathogens. In this paper the
basic technique is described and its uses and pitfalls are discussed.

INTRODUCTION

Virtually all biochemical investigations rely on the application of
alternate cycles of separation and analysis. The current dominance of
electrophoretic separations in gels for the analysis of biological macro-
molecules is due to the efficiency with which these two stages can be combined in techniques which provide both excellent resolution and easy comparison of multiple samples. However, the entrapment of the separate
components of the samples in the gel which allows great ease of handling
unfortunately precludes the use of the two most specific analytical techniques, nucleic acid hybridisation and reaction with antibodies. This
problem was solved by Southern (1975) who showed that DNA fragments resolved in agarose gels could be transferred by capillary flow to sheets of
nitrocellulose with essentially no loss of resolution. This basic idea of
high fidelity transfer to a solid phase support was then extended to RNA
and protein with the introduction of 'Northern' (Alwine et al., 1977) and
'Western' (Towbin et al., 1979; Symington et al., 1981; Burnette, 1981)
blotting. The impact of this simple but elegant analytical method in nucleic acid biochemistry has been considerable and it is clear from the frequency with which protein blots have begun to appear in the literature that
it is an important innovation which will be of particular use in the study
of microbial pathogens.

There are already a considerable number of variations in blotting
techniques and these have been reviewed recently by Gershoni and Palade
(1983). What we describe below is a technique based on that of Burnette
(1981) which we have found successful. We will attempt to draw attention

to those details which we have found important but wish to emphasise that
'Western' blotting is essentially a simple and reliable method.

THE METHOD

Blotting experiments take place in three phases, first, the separation
of the antigen mixture in a gel, usually by discontinuous SDS electrophoresis in polyacrylamide (SDS-PAGE), secondly, transfer which, with proteins, is also usually performed by electrophoresis (electroblotting) and
finally detection, in which the immobilised antigens are reacted with antibodies and the reacting species detected by a range of conventional immunological methods.

The first stage, SDS-PAGE, is now a standard technique which, for
those requiring an introduction, has been very well described by Hames
(1981). The most popular variant of the method, and the one we use, is
that described by Laemmli (1970). The protein samples are prepared for
electrophoresis by boiling for 90 secs in 'sample buffer' containing 2%
w/v SDS in 63 mM Tris pH 6.8 containing 5% v/v β-mercaptoethanol. Omission
of the last reagent allows retention of disulphide bonds but may lead to
loss of resolution of some viral polypeptides (Bastardo et al., 1981).

The gel may be loaded in two ways. For experiments in which several
antigen preparations are to be reacted with a single antiserum, the samples are loaded into wells formed with a comb in the normal way. In experiments where it is desired to test a number of different sera with a single
antigenic mixture the gel is best cast with a single large well and the
subsequent blot processed as a number of strips.

The amount of sample loaded depends on the protein complexity of the
antigen. The approximate upper capacity of the gel for a complex mixture
is 5 μg/mm^2 of sample well area. A purified virion preparation which contains a low number of polypeptide components may well require a reduced
loading.

The conditions we routinely use are as follows. Gel dimensions are
140 mm wide, 160 mm long and 0.75 mm thick (1.5 mm thick gels have also
been blotted successfully). Gel concentration is 10% with a 3% stacking
gel. The gels are run under constant current conditions at a current
density of 19 mA/cm^2 for 2-2½ hrs until the marker dye front has migrated
9 cm into the separating gel.

Electroblotting is then carried out by placing the gel (with stacking gel removed) in a sandwich consisting of filter paper (Whatmann 3 MM), a nitrocellulose sheet (Schleicher and Schull BA 83, pore size 0.2 µM), the gel and a further sheet of filter paper. This sandwich is best assembled by liberally wetting the filter paper and nitrocellulose membrane with blotting buffer and then placing the gel onto the surface of the membrane. This allows the elimination of bubbles between the gel and the membrane by gentle pressure with a gloved finger. Bubbles are the major cause of poor transfer of polypeptides to the membrane. It also allows the gel position, the position of the tracks and the position of the dye front to be marked on the membrane using a ball point pen (see Figure 1). The sandwich is then completed with a further layer of wet filter paper and mounted in the electroblotting cell with the gel towards the cathode. Many different blotting times appear in the literature but we prefer to transfer over-night at a current density of 1.3 mA/cm^2 and a voltage gradient of about 7.0 volts/cm. The blotting buffer is 20 mM Tris 154 mM glycine pH 8.3 containing 20% v/v methanol.

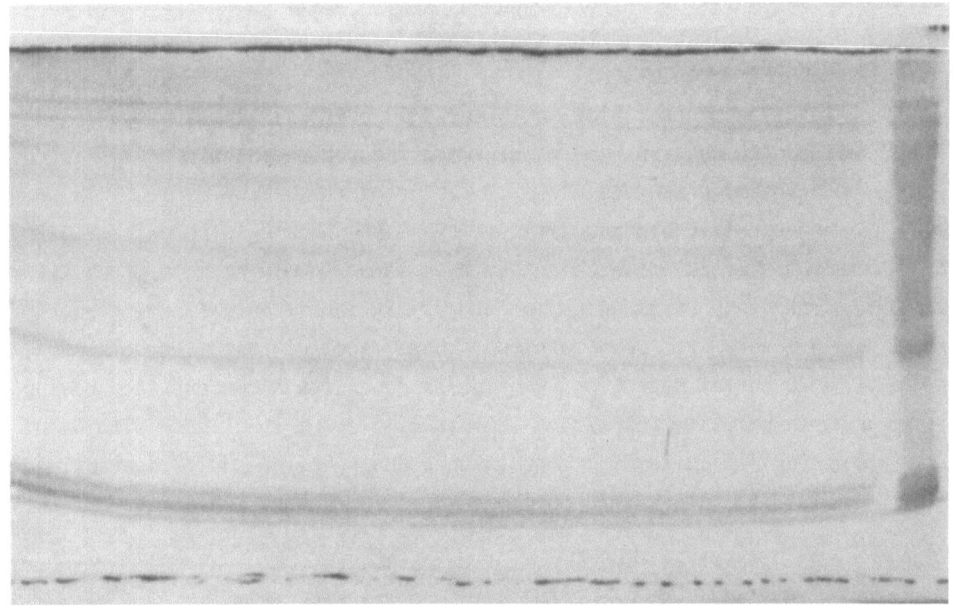

Fig.1 A stained blot to illustrate the fidelity of electrophoretic transfer. Standard proteins were run in both the main spot and the side 'standards' track. These were β-galactosidase (130K), phos-phorylase A (94K) ovotransferrin (77K) albumin (66K), ovalbumin (45K), chymotrypsinogen A (26K), myoglobin (17K) and cytochrome C (12K).

After transfer the blot is trimmed and, if necessary, cut into strips for reaction with several sera. Dry nitrocellulose membranes are prone to cracking but can be cut easily whilst damp with a sharp scalpel if placed between sheets of polythene. This also allows guidelines to be used without marking the membrane.

Staining the blot is useful for monitoring the fidelity of transfer, for displaying the polypeptide components of the antigen mixture and for the calculation of molecular weights by reference to standard proteins. The excellent fidelity of transfer achieved is illustrated in Figure 1 which shows standard proteins both in the main well and 'standards' well transferred to a membrane and stained with coomassie blue. Many of the published staining methods lead to shrinking of the membrane during staining making it difficult to relate the stained and immunoreacted blots. This problem may be overcome by staining the blot with a dilute solution of coomassie blue (16 μg/ml) in 30% methanol and 5% acetic acid. The bands appear in about 30 mins and destaining is unnecessary. Blots stained in this way may be reacted subsequently with antiserum but some bands show reduced reactivity and the staining fades during the repeated washings.

The reaction of the 'blot' with serum is performed in five stages and during all the incubations and washes described below the blot is agitated gently on a rotary shaker.

(1) The non-specific binding sites in the membrane are 'blanked' out using 50% v/v serum. It is preferable that this serum should be homologous with the final detecting serum which in our case is rabbit but we have used horse and pig sera with good results. Where labelled staphylococcal protein 'A' is used for detection blanking is done with a concentrated bovine serum albumin solution (5% w/v). The blanking serum is diluted with washing buffer (WB) which is 8.7 mM sodium phosphate buffer pH 7.2 containing 500 mM NaCl, 0.5% 'Tween 80' and 1.0 mM EDTA. Blanking is carried out for one hour at 37°C.

(2) The blot is then transferred to the test serum and incubated for a further hour at room temperature. The test serum is typically diluted 1:50 in 10% v/v blanking serum in WB.

(3) The next stage is a thorough wash in WB without serum. Washing consists of three rapid rinses followed by three 5 minute washes followed by three more rapid rinses.

(4) The blot is now incubated in the detection serum diluted in 10% blanking serum in WB for 1 hr at room temperature. Our detection antibody is an affinity column purified rabbit anti-sheep Fab_2 IgG which we iodinate to a specific activity of 3 x 10^5 cpm/μg and use a dilution of around 4 x 10^5 cpm/ml. (Typically 2 mg of this IgG are reacted with 1 mCi of ^{125}I in the chloramine T reaction (Hunter and Greenwood, 1962). This iodinated antibody has been found to have a useful life of up to 4 months.

(5) After incubation the filters are given a further thorough wash as described above and are vacuum dried and mounted on filter paper for autoradiography. This is performed using overnight exposure to Kodak X omat 'S' film with a Dupont 'lightening plus' intensifying screen.

Apparatus for blotting is available from 'EC' corporation St., Petersburg, Florida, or from Biorad, Richmond, California. 'Homemade' blotting cells also appear to give good results (Towbin et al., 1979).

PITFALLS AND INTERPRETATION OF RESULTS

A positive result in a 'Western' blot indicates that the detection serum has bound to a band but unfortunately this does not always indicate that a specific immune reaction has occurred between the protein in the band and antibodies in the test serum. We have observed a variety of non-specific reactions which can be recognised by using control incubations. The most common form of non-specific reaction is the binding of immunoglobulins in the test serum to denatured proteins on the blot probably through hydrophobic interactions. This can be detected by the inclusion of control sera either from pre-bleeds or from non-immune animals preferably age matched with the immune sera donors. Non-specific binding is usually much weaker than genuine immune reactions.

It is appropriate at this point to mention the central disadvantage of 'Western' blotting from SDS-polyacrylamide gels which is that the proteins which are used as antigens are denatured at the start of the procedure and this destroys many antigenic determinants which are conformational in nature and exposes the hydrophobic domains present in many proteins. Some renaturation of the protein may occur on the membrane surface but the majority of determinants detected will be those which depend solely on the primary structure of the polypeptide chains. It is thus not surprising that highly structural antigens such as non-enveloped viruses do not appear to generate many antibodies directed against these sequential determinants unless purified viral proteins are used as antigens. Enveloped viruses and complex prokaryotic pathogens, however, appear to generate many such antibodies. Indeed, in the case of complex antigenic pathogens 'Western' blotting has the advantage of simplifying the analysis of the immune response. It also has the advantage that since no pathogens are known which can withstand boiling in SDS and mercaptoethanol the method can be safely used to compare viral antigens from different parts of the world without the need to transport live virus.

In addition to non-specific binding to proteins other effects may be observed. Many blots show diffuse bands with apparent molecular weights of about 50 K. These are caused by non-specific binding to substances present in the mercaptoethanol in the sample buffer which can be readily detected in the gel by silver staining (Tasheva and Dessev, 1983) and which are transferred to the membrane. These bands are not seen when proteins are present in this region of the gel. Another type of false positive was reported by Newhall et al. (1982) who found positive reactions to venereal-ly transmitted strains of Chlamydia trachomatis with the sera of cloister-ed nuns and children. Subsequently it was found that two proteins of cer-tain C. trachomatis strains had the ability to bind human immunoglobulins but not those of other species. Specific reactions were observed with other chlamydial antigens.

THE USE OF PROTEIN BLOTTING IN VIRAL DIAGNOSIS

The vast majority of blotting applications reported to date have been in the field of microbiological research and the technique has not yet found a place in routine diagnosis. However, blotting has a major role to play in the development of the coming generation of diagnostic tests and is useful for certain low scale routine applications.

An example of a low scale use for blotting is the test we have recent-ly developed to detect a retrovirus which we believe is the aetiological agent of sheep pulmonary adenomatosis (SPA, also called jaagsiekte) in lung exudates and tumour homogenates. Initially this virus was detected by electron microscopy (Perk et al., 1971) and subsequently its presence in lung tumours and homogenates was confirmed by the demonstration of a particle associated reverse transcriptase activity (Perk et al., 1974; Herring et al., 1983). Recently (Sharp and Herring, 1983) we have shown that the virus can be sensitively detected in lung exudates and tumour homogenates from both field cases and experimentally infected sheep using blotted antigens and a hyperimmune goat serum raised against the core (gag) protein of a type D retrovirus, Mason Pfizer monkey virus. The positive reaction is with a protein of 25K as shown in Figure 2; this is typical of the size of retroviral major core proteins. Recently we have used this test to show the presence of the SPA retrovirus in lung exudates from sheep from Peru and South Africa (unpublished results).

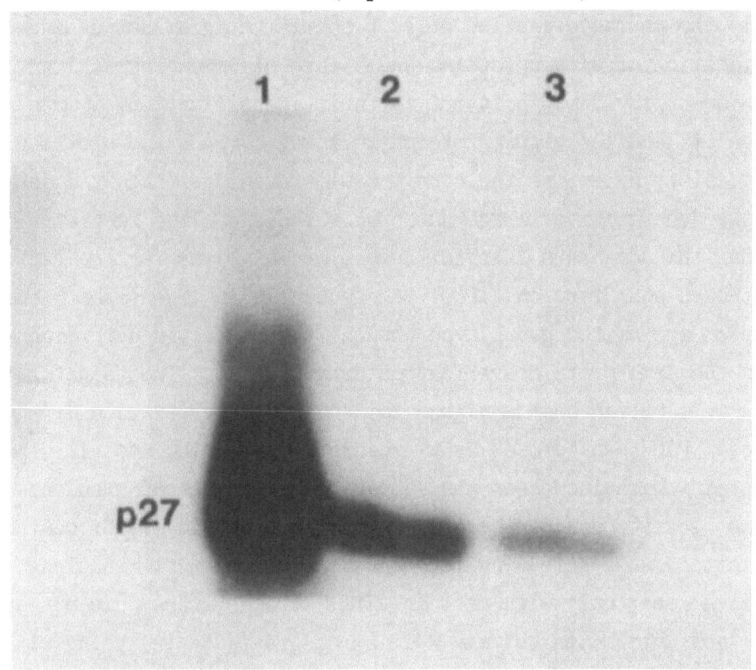

Fig. 2   Blotted proteins from   1. Mason Pfizer monkey virus.
2. SPA retrovirus and 3. Mouse mammary tumour virus reacted with
a hyperimmune goat antiserum to Mason Pfizer monkey virus p27.

It is interesting that the lung exudates which contain the SPA retrovirus also contain substantial amounts of immunoglobulins, especially IgA. This considerably complicates the detection of viral antigens by any other type of indirect test but, fortunately, the viral antigen, p25, is separated in the gel from immunoglobulin light chain which does react weakly with our detection serum. Blotting has thus provided the first practical detection system for this virus but, unfortunately, infected sheep do not produce detectable antibodies to SDS denatured p25. Thus our primary aim of producing a serological screening test for the disease will have to await the further identification of the other protein components of the virus.

It is notable that the detection system described above depends on
the presence of group antigens common to the SPA retrovirus, Mason-Pfizer
monkey virus and mouse mammary tumour virus. With the advent of monoclonal
antibodies such group antigens have assumed considerable importance since
they, rather than more restricted type specific antigens, are the determinants of choice for tests to achieve the initial identification of virus.
Previously the characterisation of such shared antigens has depended on
the purification of viral proteins and a careful immunochemical analysis.
Two techniques provide a short cut to their identification, immune precipitation of labelled virus proteins followed by PAGE and blotting. Of
these two, blotting enjoys the considerable advantage that it does not
require the generation of large numbers of radiolabelled samples. Indeed,
it also has the advantage that for some types of virus (eg the retroviridae
see Versteegen and Oroszlan, 1980) the sequential antigens which survive
denaturation are of the group type whereas type specific determinants contained in the same protein are lost on denaturation. Thus denatured proteins may well be the best antigens to use for the generation of monoclonal
antibodies. PAGE can be used as a preparative technique to yield purified
virus protein which increases considerably the chances of a successful
fusion and blotting can be used as a screening technique. Of course, the
use of blotting as a screening technique may also reveal monoclonal reagents which react only with certain viral strains, these are not appropriate detection antibodies but may well be of great use in typing virus.

Blotting can also be used for serological diagnosis and studies using
blotting may well yield useful clues about the viral antigens which elicit
the earliest and the strongest humoural responses; information which is
most important in the design of serological screens. A technique for
assaying antibody which is related to blotting also deserves mention; this
is 'dot-blotting' in which the antigen is simply spotted onto the nitrocellulose membrane (Hawkes et al., 1982). This technique is a valuable
alternative to ELISA, especially for small scale applications, since most
antigens bind tenaciously to nitrocellulose and the uncertainties of the
plate binding step are avoided.

To conclude, blotting is a simple and fairly quick technique which
appends the powerful resolution of SDS-PAGE to 'traditional' solid-phase
technique. Currently we are using the technique to identify antigens in a

paramyxovirus, two retroviruses and several pestiviruses and have obtained successful preliminary results with mycoplasmas, chlamydia and toxoplasma. It represents a powerful weapon in the virologist's armoury and we commend it wholeheartedly.

REFERENCES

Alwine, J.C., Kemp, D.J. and Stark, G.R. 1977. Method for detection of specific RNAs in agarose gels by transfer to DBM paper and hybridisation with DNA probes. Proc. Natl. Acad. Sci. USA, 74, 5350-5354.

Bastardo, J.W., McKimm-Breschkin, J.L., Sonza, S., Mercer, L.D. and Holmes, I.H. 1981. Preparation and characterisation of antisera to electrophoretically purified SA11 virus polypeptides. Infect. Immun., 34, 641-647.

Burnette, W.N. 1981. 'Western Blotting': electrophoretic transfer of proteins from SDS-polyacrylamide gels to unmodified nitrocellulose and radiographic detection with antibody and radioiodinated protein A. Anal. Biochem., 112, 195-203.

Gershoni, J.M. and Palade, G.E. 1983. Protein Blotting: principles and applications. Anal. Biochem., 131, 1-15.

Hames, B.D. 1981. In "Gel electrophoresis of proteins" (Ed. B.D. Hames and D. Rickwood). (IRL Press, Oxford and Washington DC).

Hawkes, R., Niday, E. and Gordon, J. 1982. A Dot-immunobinding assay for monoclonal and other antibodies. Anal. Biochem., 119, 142-147.

Herring, A.J., Sharp, J.M., Scott, F.M.M. and Angus, K.W. 1983. Further evidence for a retrovirus as the aetiological agent of sheep pulmonary adenomatosis (jaagsiekte). Vet. Microbiol., 8, 237-249.

Hunter, W.M. and Greenwood, F.C. 1962. Preparation of iodine-131 labelled human growth hormone of high specific activity. Nature, 194, 495-496.

Laemmli, U.K. 1970. Cleavage of structural proteins during the assembly of the head of bacteriophage T4. Nature, 227, 680-685.

Newhall, W.J., Batteiger, B. and Jones, R.G. 1982. Analysis of the human serological response to proteins of Chlamydia trachomatis. Infect. Immun., 38, 1181-1189.

Perk, K., Hod, I. and Nobel, T.A. 1971. Pulmonary adenomatosis of sheep (jaagsiekte). 1. Ultrastructure of the tumour. J. Natl. Cancer Inst., 4, 525-537.

Perk, K., Michalides, R., Spiegelman, S. and Schlom, J. 1974. Biochemical and morphologic evidence for the presence of RNA tumour virus in pulmonary carcinoma of sheep (jaagsiekte). J. Natl. Cancer Inst., 53, 131-135.

Sharp, J.M. and Herring, A.J. 1983. Sheep pulmonary adenomatosis: demonstration of a protein which cross reacts with the major core proteins of Mason-Pfizer monkey virus and mouse mammary tumour virus. J. gen. Virol., 64, 2323-2327.

Southern, E.M. 1975. Detection of specific sequences among DNA fragments separated by gel electrophoresis. J. Mol. Biol., 98, 503-517.

Symington, J., Green, M. and Brackmann, K. 1981. Immunoautoradiographic detection of proteins after electrophoretic transfer from gels to diazopaper: analysis of adenovirus encoded proteins. Proc. Natl. Acad. Sci. USA, 78, 177-181.

Tasheva, B. and Dessev, G. 1983. Artifacts in SDS-polyacrylamide gel electrophoresis due to 2-mercaptoethanol. Anal. Biochem., 129, 98-102.

Towbin, J., Staehelin, T. and Gordon, J. 1979. Electrophoretic transfer of proteins from polyacrylamide gels to nitrocellulose sheets: procedure and some applications. Proc. Natl. Acad. Sci. USA, 76, 4350-4354.

Versteegen, R.J. and Oroszlan, S. 1980. Effect of chemical modification and fragmentation on antigenic determinants of internal protein p30 and surface protein gp70 of type C retroviruses. J. Virol., 33, 983-992.

THE USE OF POLYACRYLAMIDE GEL ELECTROPHORESIS OF VIRUS RNA
IN THE STUDY OF ROTAVIRUS INFECTIONS

D. Todd, M.S. McNulty, G.M. Allan

Veterinary Research Laboratories
Stormont, Belfast BT4 3SD, N. Ireland

ABSTRACT

Polyacrylamide gel electrophoresis of rotavirus RNA has been used to provide diagnostically and epidemiologically useful information about avian and mammalian rotavirus infections. (1) Rotaviruses possessing four different electropherotypes were detected in a longitudinal survey of a 34,000 bird broiler flock. Two of these had not been described previously in chickens. When virus recognisates were grouped according to electropherotype, infection with different electropherotypes was seen to occur in waves, with each wave lasting about one week. Cross-immunofluorescence indicated that rotaviruses with different electropherotypes were antigenically distinct, with only one sharing an antigen with conventional mammalian rotaviruses. (2) Much intra-species variation was observed when bovine and porcine rotavirus RNAs obtained from different farms were analysed on high resolution 12.5% polyacrylamide gels. Consistent differences were observed between bovine and porcine rotavirus RNA profiles. The detection of additional bands in some RNA profiles indicated that more than one population of rotavirus was present in some faeces specimens. The finding that only one electropherotype was observed in samples taken from heifer calves from a "closed" dairy farm over a 16 month period suggested that only one rotavirus was present and that its genome was electrophoretically stable. (3) One electrophoretically "atypical" recognisate was observed out of 70 samples from bovine or porcine clinical cases.

INTRODUCTION

Rotavirus infections have been associated with neonatal enteritis in a wide variety of animal species (McNulty, 1978). They are commonly diagnosed by electron microscopic examination (Madeley et al., 1977) or enzymelinked immunoassay (Grauballe et al., 1981) of faeces samples.

The genome of mammalian and avian rotaviruses consists of 11 segments of double-stranded RNA which can be separated by polyacrylamide gel electrophoresis (PAGE) and range in mol. wt. from about 2.0×10^6 to 0.2×10^6 (Kalica et al., 1978; Todd et al., 1980). Electrophoretic analysis of rotavirus RNA extracted from faeces has been used in diagnosis (Herring et al., 1982), and since differences in the migration pattern of individual RNA segments have allowed strains to be distinguished, also as a tool for studying rotavirus epidemiology (Rodger et al., 1981; Schnagl et al., 1981; Follett and Desselberger, 1983).

In this report we describe how PAGE has been of use diagnostically and epidemiologically in our studies of rotavirus infections in chickens, cattle and pigs.

MATERIALS AND METHODS

Faeces samples

In a detailed survey of a 34,000 bird broiler flock, twelve birds were usually removed twice weekly and their gut contents collected. Samples of bovine and porcine faeces were obtained from clinical outbreaks of diarrhoea.

Electron microscopy

Examination of faecal material was carried out as described for method C of McNulty et al. (1979) except that the final pelleting of the virus was carried out in an Eppendorf model 5414 centrifuge at 12,500 g for 15 minutes.

Immunofluorescence

Cross immunofluorescence tests were performed using infected primary chick embryo liver (CEL) cells or embryo rhesus monkey kidney (MA104) cells infected with the appropriate rotaviruses and sera from experimentally infected chickens as described by McNulty et al. (1984).

Preparation of RNA from faeces

Five or 10% faeces suspensions in phosphate buffered saline (PBS) were sonicated, treated with sodium dodecyl sulphate (SDS) at a final concentration of 0.25% and extracted with the fluorcarbon Arcton 113 (ICI Ltd., Runcorn, England). The clarified extract was centrifuged at 110,000 g for 1.5 h at $20^{\circ}C$ through a 2 ml cushion of 30% (w/w) sucrose using a 6 x 14 ml swing-out rotor. The crude virus pellet was resuspended in 0.1 M sodium acetate-acetic acid pH 5.0 (acetate) buffer containing 1% SDS and extracted twice with phenol and once with chloroform/isoamyl alcohol. Following precipitation with ethanol, virus RNA was dissolved in 50 µl of acetate buffer containing 0.1 µg/ml Ribonuclease A (Sigma) and 20 µg/ml Deoxyribonuclease (Sigma) and incubated for 0.5 h at $37^{\circ}C$. Samples were prepared for electrophoresis by the addition of an equal volume of 30% sucrose in electrophoresis buffer.

Polyacrylamide gel electrophoresis

Gels containing 5% acrylamide were prepared and electrophoresed as described previously (Todd et al., 1980). Gels containing 12.5% acrylamide were prepared using a modification of the method published by Marsden et al. (1978). The 5% stacking gel was prepared in 0.122 M Tris - HCl, pH 6.7 containing 0.1% SDS and the resolving gel (16 cm x 14 cm) in 0.375 M Tris - HCl, pH 8.9 containing 0.1% SDS. Electrophoresis buffer contained 0.05 M Tris, 0.05 M glycine, pH 8.9 and 0.1% SDS. Samples were electrophoresed at 10 m A/gel for 40 h. Gels were stained in ethidium bromide (1 µg/ml) and photographed using a UV transilluminator.

RESULTS AND DISCUSSION

Avian rotaviruses

A detailed longitudinal survey was carried out on a 34,000 bird broiler house which was stocked with birds from several supply farms. Rotavirus was detected in the faeces of randomly selected birds by electron microscopy intermittently from 9-50 days (Table 1). RNA was extracted from

TABLE 1   Longitudinal survey of a broiler flock for rotavirus excretion: electrophoretic typing of the recognisates.

Age (days)	No. faeces in which rotavirus was detected/No. faeces examined	Electropherotype			
		1	2	3	4
9	3/12			3	
16	7/12			4	
22	1/12		1		
26	3/11	2	1		
27	2/12	1	1		
29	3/12	1	1		
36	1/12			1	
43	4/12				4
47	5/12				5
50	3/12				2

No virus detected at 5, 19, 33, 34, 41, 54, 58, 62, 65, 69 and 75 days.

all samples of gut contents in which virus was detected and electrophoresed in 5% polyacrylamide gels. Rotavirus double-stranded RNA segments were

recognised in most of these samples and it was possible to assign the rotavirus recognisates to 1 of 4 different RNA electropherotypes (Fig. 1). Between 9 and 16 days rotaviruses with electropherotype 3 predominated, between 22 and 29 days those with electropherotypes 1 and 2 were present and
between 43 and 50 days the majority of recognisates possessed electropherotype 4 (Table 1). It was apparent therefore that rotavirus infection
occurred in a series of discrete waves with each wave lasting about one
week.

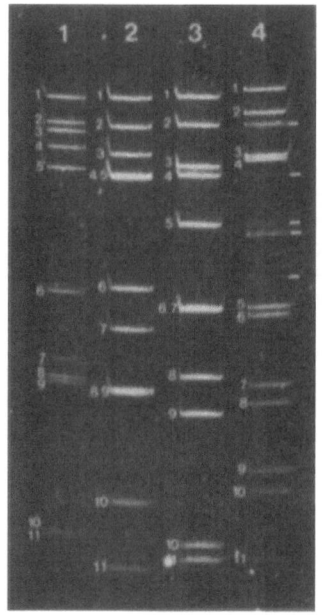

Fig. 1   Electrophoresis of avian rotavirus RNAs in a 5% polyacrylamide gel, showing profiles for electropherotypes 1, 2, 3 and
4. Unlabelled bands present in the profile of electropherotype 4
were considered to be contaminating RNA since they were absent in
other electropherotype 4 profiles and present in samples lacking
rotavirus RNA.

Electropherotypes 1 and 2 closely resembled those of the Ch1 and 132 rotavirus respectively, which had been isolated and characterised previously in this laboratory (Todd et al., 1980; McNulty et al., 1981). Ch1 rotavirus shares an antigen with the majority of mammalian rotaviruses examined to date (McNulty et al., 1980) whereas 132 rotavirus does not (McNulty et al., 1981). Electropherotypes 3 and 4 have not been previously described in chickens. One point of interest in the profiles of these electropherotypes was the separation of RNA segment 7 from segments 8 and 9 in the case of electropherotype 3 and segment 9 from segments 7 and 8 in the case of electropherotype 4. Similar splitting of the 7, 8 and 9 triplet has been observed in 132 rotavirus RNA and in all other atypical mammalian rotaviruses which lack the rotavirus group antigen shared by the majority of rotaviruses (McNulty et al., 1981; Bridger et al., 1982; Bohl et al., 1982; Nicolas et al., 1983; Rodger et al., 1982). Representative rotaviruses with electropherotype 3 (A4) and electropherotype 4 (555) were therefore investigated antigenically. Although these viruses could not be adapted to grow in tissue culture, limited growth in CEL cells and the use of sera from experimentally infected chickens allowed indirect cross-immunofluorescence tests to be performed. The results of this analysis (Table 2) provide evidence for the existence of 4 distinct antigenic subgroups of rotavirus in chickens, which do not cross-react by immunofluorescence.

TABLE 2   Antigenic relationships of chicken rotaviruses by indirect immunofluorescence.

Antiserum	Virus			
	132	Ch1	A4	555
132	>10,000*	<40	<40	< 40
Ch1	<40	>10,000	<40	< 40
A4	40	<40	640	< 40
555	<40	<40	<40	320

* Indirect immunofluorescence titre of antiserum.

Mammalian rotaviruses

This work was undertaken to investigate the diversity of bovine and porcine rotavirus RNA electropherotypes. To achieve high resolution, gels containing 12.5% acrylamide were employed (Sabara et al., 1982).

The RNA profiles shown in Fig. 2 are typical of those observed for bovine rotaviruses obtained from different farms. Such samples were rarely

130

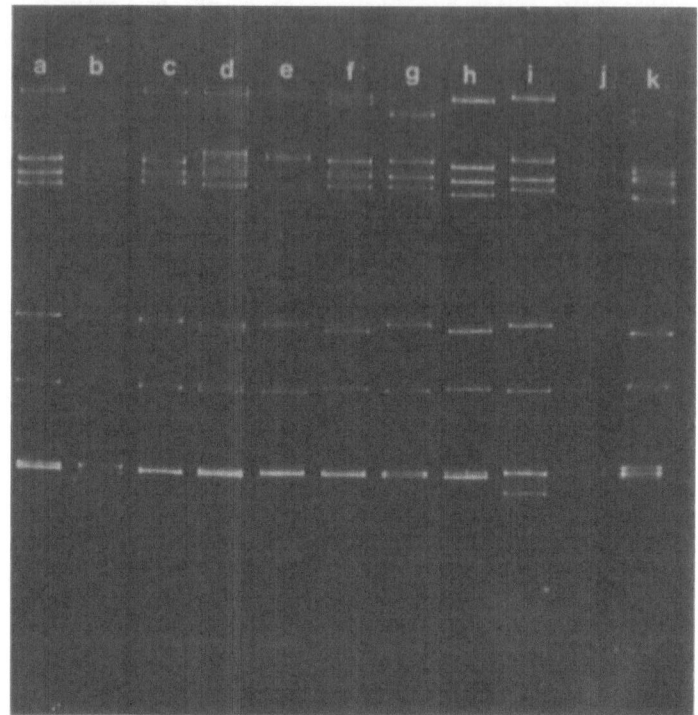

Fig. 2   Electrophoresis of bovine rotavirus RNAs in a 12.5% polyacrylamide gel. Electropherotypes a - k were obtained from different
farms.

identical by this PAGE system, with minor variations occurring in most of
the 11 segments. Samples taken from different outbreaks on the same farm
were often different (results not shown). Indeed the detection of additional bands in some faeces specimens (for example Fig. 2, d, and k) would
suggest that more than one population of rotavirus was present.

In contrast to the large electrophoretic variation observed in Fig. 2,
analysis of samples collected in a longitudinal survey of a "closed" dairy
farm (McNulty and Logan, 1983) showed that only one electropherotype was
present from November 1981 to March 1983 (Fig. 3). It seemed likely that
one rotavirus population was present and that its genome had remained
electrophoretically "stable".

Examination of pig faeces which were shown to contain rotavirus by
electron microscopy revealed similar electrophoretic variation to that observed with bovine samples (Fig. 4). Although samples from different farms
were usually different (Fig. 4, c and d) samples from different animals

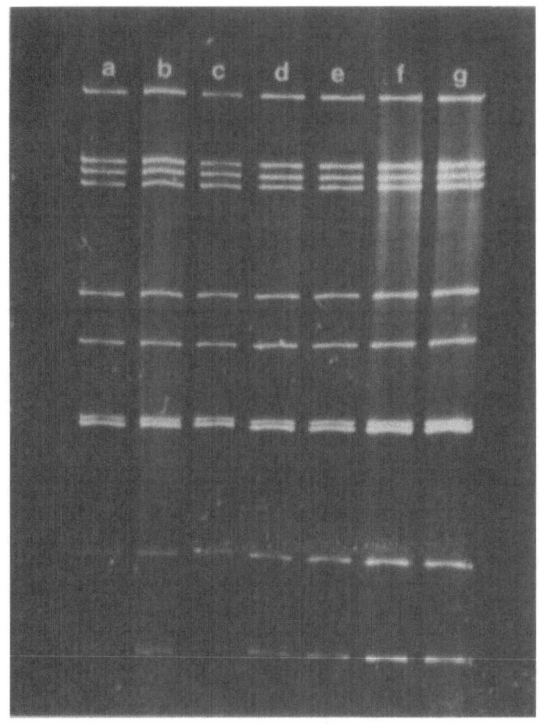

Fig 3.   Electrophoresis of bovine rotavirus RNAs in a 12.5% polyacrylamide gel. Electropherotypes a - f were obtained at different
times from November 1981 to March 1983 from one "closed" dairy farm.
Profile g represents a co-electrophoresis of samples a and f.

obtained during the same outbreak of diarrhoea were identical (Fig. 4, f
and g, h and i).

Examination of more than 25 rotavirus RNA profiles from each species
has revealed consistent differences between porcine and bovine rotavirus
RNA electropherotypes. Under these conditions of electrophoresis RNA segment 5 migrates more slowly, segments 7, 8 and 9 are more tightly bunched
and segment 11 migrates more rapidly in the calf rotavirus RNA profile
(Fig. 5).

It will be interesting to see whether these findings hold true for
every typical calf and pig rotavirus. Our results suggest, however, that
while cross-infection between these animal species is experimentally possible, its occurrence in the field is at least uncommon. This apparent
absence of cross-infection may be due to the type of husbandry practised in

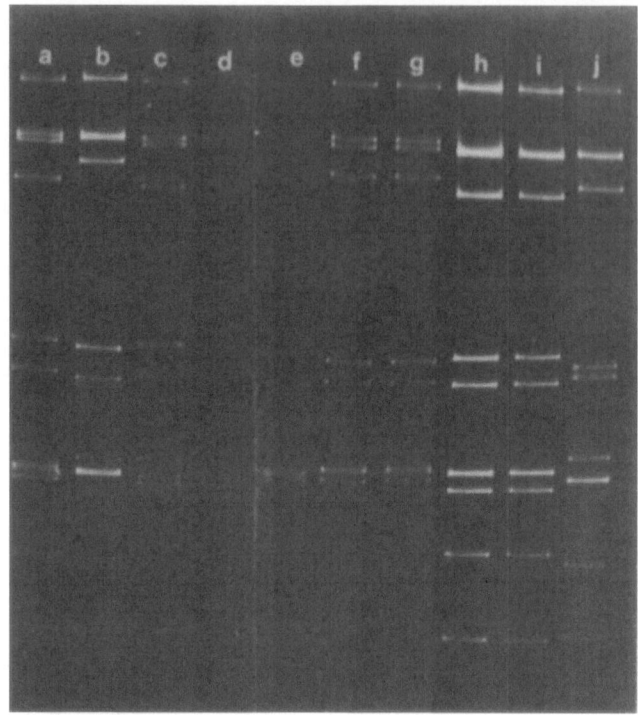

Fig. 4   Electrophoresis of porcine rotavirus RNAs in a 12.5% polyacrylamide gel. Electropherotypes a - j were obtained from different
clinical specimens.

Northern Ireland where the vast majority of pigs are intensively farmed and
therefore separated from cattle.

One of the reasons for undertaking this work was to look for "atypical"
mammalian rotaviruses. Examination of porcine and bovine faeces which were
positive by electron microscopy yielded one possible candidate out of 70
samples (Fig. 6). Shortage of material and its failure to grow in cell
culture or in experimentally infected calves have prevented us from obtaining a better RNA profile. The separation of RNA segment 9 from segments 7
and 8 and the close migration of 5 and 6 is unusual and indeed bears a
strong resemblance to Type B RNA profiles published by Pedley et al. (1983).
It is difficult to assess the prevalence and economic importance of
atypical mammalian rotaviruses in Northern Ireland. It must be remembered
that if these viruses frequently cause asymptomatic infection, the samples
we receive from clinical cases may not be the most suitable for their detection.

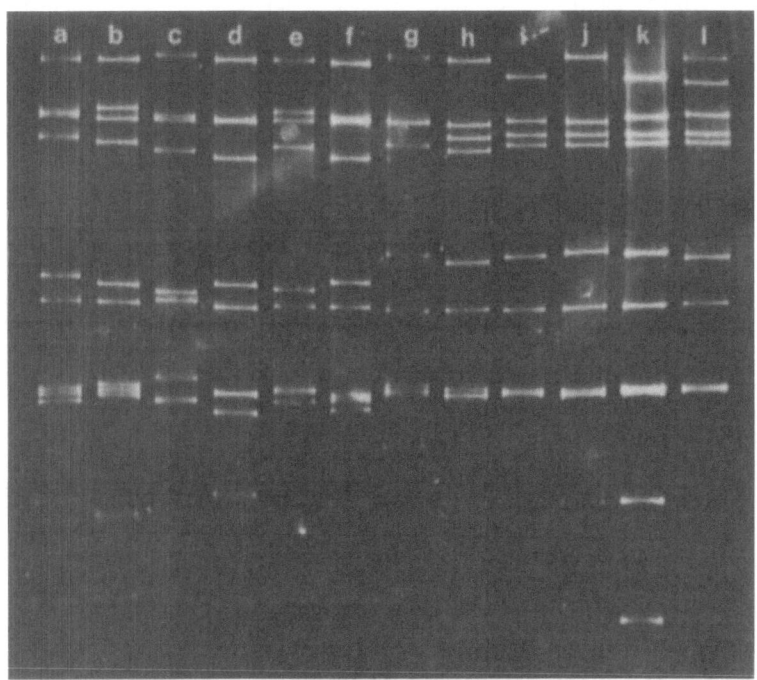

Fig. 5   Electrophoresis of porcine and bovine rotavirus RNAs in a 12.5% polyacrylamide gel. Electropherotypes a - f and g - 1 were obtained from representative porcine and bovine samples respectively.

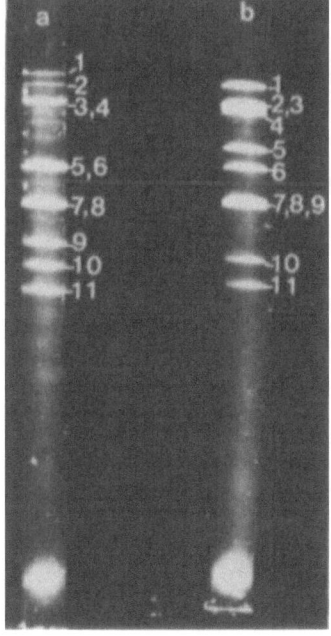

134

Fig. 6   Electrophoresis of bovine rotavirus RNAs in 5% cylindinal
polyacrylamide gels. Electropherotype b is a typical bovine rotavirus
RNA profile whereas electropherotype a possibly belongs to an atypical
bovine rotavirus.

REFERENCES

Bohl, E.H., Saif, L.J., Theil, K.W., Agnes, A.G. and Cross, R.F. 1982.
    Porcine pararotavirus: detection, differentiation from rotavirus and
    pathogenesis in gnotobiotic piglets. J. Clin. Microbiol., 15, 312-
    319.
Bridger, J.C., Clarke, I.N. and McCrae, M.A. 1982. Characterisation of an
    antigenically distinct porcine rotavirus. Infect. Immun., 35, 1058-
    1062.
Follett, E.A.C. and Desselberger, U. 1983. Co-circulation of different
    rotavirus strains in a local outbreak of infantile gastroenteritis:
    monitoring by rapid and sensitive nucleic acid analysis. J. Med.
    Virol., 11, 39-52.
Grauballe, P.C., Vestergaard, B.F., Meyling, A. and Genner, J. 1981. Op-
    timized enzyme-linked immunosorbent assay for detection of human and
    bovine rotavirus in stools: Comparison with electron microscopy,
    immunoelectro-osmophoresis and fluorescent antibody techniques. J.
    Med. Virol., 7, 29-40.
Herring, A.J., Inglis, N.F., Ojeh, C.K., Snodgrass, D.R. and Menzies, J.D.
    1982. Rapid diagnosis of rotavirus infection by direct detection of
    vial nucleic acid in silver-stained polyacrylamide gels. J. Clin.
    Microbiol., 16, 473-477.
Kalica, A.R., Wyatt, R.G. and Kapikian, A.Z. 1978. Detection of differences
    among human and animal rotavirus using analysis of viral RNA. J. Am.
    Vet. Med. Assoc., 173, 531-537.
Madeley, C.R., Cosgrove, B.P., Bell, E.J. and Fallon, R.J. 1977. Stool
    viruses in babies in Glasgow. 1. Hospital admissions with diar-
    rhoea. J. Hyg. (Cambridge), 78, 261-273.
Marsden, H.S., Stow, N.D., Preston, V.G., Timbury, M.C. and Wilkie, N.M.
    1978. Physical mapping of herpesvirus - induced polypeptides. J.
    Virol., 28, 624-642.
McNulty, M.S. 1978. Rotaviruses. J. Gen. Virol., 40, 1-18.
McNulty, M.S., Curran, W.L., Todd, D. and McFerran, J.B. 1979. Detection
    of viruses in avian faeces by direct electron microscopy. Avian.
    Pathol., 8,239-247.
McNulty, M.S., Allan, G.M., Todd, D., McFerran, J.B., McKillop, E.R.,
    Collins, D.S. and McCracken, R.M. 1980. Isolation of rotaviruses from
    turkeys and chickens: demonstration of distinct serotypes and electro-
    pherotypes. Avian. Pathol., 9, 363-375.
McNulty, M.S., Allan, G.M., Todd, D., McFerran, J.B. and McCracken, R.M.
    1981. Isolation from chickens of a rotavirus lacking the rotavirus
    group antigen. J. Gen. Virol., 55, 405-413.
McNulty, M.S. and Logan, E.F. 1983. Longitudinal survey of rotavirus in-
    fection in calves. Vet. Rec., 113, 333-335.
McNulty, M.S., Todd, D., Allan, G.M., McFerran, J.B. and Greene, J.A. 1984.
    Epidemiology of rotavirus infection in broiler chickens. Arch.
    Virol.,
Nicolas, J.C., Cohen, J., Fortier, B., Lourenco, M.H. and Bricout, F. 1983.
    Isolation of a human pararotavirus. Virol., 124, 181-184.

Pedley, S., Bridger, J.C., Brown, J.F. and McCrae, M.A. 1983. Molecular characterisation of rotaviruses with distinct group antigens. J. Gen. Virol., 64,

Rodger, S.M., Bishop, R.F., Birch, C., McLean, B. and Holmes, I.H. 1981. Molecular epidemiology of human rotaviruses in Melbourne, Australia from 1973 to 1979, as determined by electrophoresis of genome ribonucleic acid. J. Clin. Microbiol., 13, 272-278.

Rodger, S.M., Bishop, R.F. and Holmes, I.H. 1982. Detection of a rotavirus-like agent associated with diarrhoea in an infant. J. Clin. Microbiol. 724-726.

Schnagl, R.D., Rodger, S.M. and Holmes, I.H. 1981. Variation in human rotavirus electropherotypes occurring between rotavirus gastroenteritis epidemics in Central Australia. Infect. Immun., 33, 17-21.

Sabara, M., Deregt, D., Babiuk, L. and Misra, V. 1982. Genetic heterogeneity within individual bovine rotavirus isolates. J. Virol., 44, 813-822.

Todd, D., McNulty, M.S. and Allan, G.M. 1980. Polyacrylamide gel electrophoresis of avian rotavirus RNA. Arch. Virol., 63, 87-97.

EXAMINATION OF ROTAVIRUS FROM BOVINE AND PORCINE SPECIES
BY WESTERN BLOTTING

Anette G. Boetner and Jon Askaa

Department of Veterinary Virology and Immunology,
The Royal Veterinary and Agricultural University of Copenhagen,
Bulowsvej 13, 1870 Copenhagen V, Denmark.

ABSTRACT

The "Western blotting technique" has been applied to rotavirus isolates from bovine and porcine species. Five to six polypeptides were identified for both bovine and porcine rotavirus with estimated molecular
weights (MW) of 150-160K, 140-145K, 99K, 60-65K, 40-49K and 30K, of which
the 40-49K polypeptide band was the strongest. These results were obtained
when the virus samples were dissociated by immersing in boiling water for
3 mins before SDS-PAGE. When the virus samples were heated for 10 mins at
56°C instead, a total dissociation of the virus proteins did not occur and
only two polypeptides with estimated MW of 80-85K and 95-100K appeared, of
which the 80-85K polypeptide was the most intense. The possibility that
the 80-85K polypeptide consists partly of the 40-49K polypeptide is discussed.

INTRODUCTION

Electrophoretic transfer of polypeptides from sodium dodecyl sulfate-
polyacrylamide gel electrophoresis (SDS-PAGE) gels to untreated nitrocellulose sheets has been called "Western blotting" (Towbin et al., 1979;
Burnette, 1981). On the basis of their antigenicity the transferred polypeptides can be identified on the nitrocellulose sheet by the use of radioactive or enzyme labelled antibodies. When virus specific antibodies are
used for the blotting technique only the virus specific bands will appear.
Hereby elaborate virus purification procedures can be avoided. Until
recently the majority of all rotavirus isolates have been found to contain
a common group antigen, but species specific antigens have also been demonstrated. The virus antigens have been demonstrated using SDS-PAGE on
purified virus, crossed immunoelectrophoresis, serum neutralisation tests
and plaque reduction assay (Flewett et al., 1974; Woode et al., 1976;
Grauballe et al., 1977; Novo and Esparza, 1981; Estes and Graham, 1980).

Application of the "Western blotting technique" to rotavirus isolates
from bovine and porcine species might demonstrate differences between these
isolates and maybe among serotypes too. In the following experiments we
attempted to establish the "Western blotting technique" with rotavirus isolates, and to identify and compare the bands obtained.

MATERIALS AND METHODS

Preparation of antigens

Faeces samples were collected from calves and piglets with diarrhoea originating from different farms in Denmark. Each faeces sample was ground in Eagle's essential medium (Gibco) containing penicillin and dihydro-streptomycin to make a 20% faecal suspension. After low speed centrifugation (2000 x g for 20 mins) the supernatant were stored at -40°C until further processing or examination.

A portion of the supernatant was homogenized with 10% FREON (trichloro-trifluor-ethane) on a sonic disintegrator (model 300 ARTEK) and centrifuged at 2000 x g for 20 mins. The resultant aqueous phase was collected (FREON faeces, FF) and stored at -40°C.

Rotavirus was isolated from faeces samples by inoculation of a fetal monkey kidney cell line (MA 104) (kindly provided by Dr E.H. Bohl, O.A.R.D.C., Ohio). The cells were grown to a confluent monolayer in a medium containing 10% normal calf serum. Before inoculation cells were washed three times in medium without serum. The faeces supernatant was treated with trypsin (Difco trypsin 1:250) at a concentration of 100 µg/ml for one hour at 37°C before inoculation into cell cultures. The trypsin treated suspension was diluted tenfold in Eagle's essential medium, and the dilution was absorbed for one hour on a confluent cell monolayer. After absorption the inoculum was discarded, and a maintenance medium containing 0.5% bovine serum albumin and 0.5-1 µg trypsin per ml was added. The cells were observed in the microscope throughout the experimental period for development of cytopathologic changes. Three to six days after inoculation the cell cultures were frozen. Before passage of the harvests to new cell cultures the cells were frozen and thawed three times. The harvests were passed to new confluent monolayer cultures after treatment of the harvest with 10 µg trypsin per ml for one hour at 37°C.

Supernatants from faeces suspensions as well as the different preparations of the cell culture harvests were tested for rotavirus group antigen by a commercially available ELISA system (DAKOPATTS a/s, Denmark described by Askaa and Bloch, 1981 and Grauballe et al., 1981). Both faeces samples and cell culture harvests with and without rotavirus antigen were included in the examinations.

Purification of rotavirus propagated in cell culture

Harvests from cell cultures were clarified by low speed centrifugation.

This low speed centrifuged virus suspension (LSV) was ultrafiltered through
a Diaflo ultrafilter XM100A (Amicon) to a final volume of 1/7 of the original volume (the concentrate was washed with 0.9% sodium chloride) (concentrated virus, CV). Immunosorbent chromatography was used for purification of virus used for immunization of rabbits. Carbonyl groups were
introduced into Sepharose 6B according to Shainoff (1980). IgG from a
bovine rotavirus hyperimmune serum was purified by passage over a protein A
column and the IgG was coupled to the carbonyl activated Sepharose by the
addition of sodium cyanoborohydride (Shainoff, 1980). The LSV was added to
the column, and the antibody-bound protein was eluted with citric acid,
pH 3.

Antisera

A bovine convalescent serum was obtained from a calf 10 days after it
was found to excrete rotavirus antigen in faeces.

Two antigen preparations were used for hyperimmunization of rabbits.
These were a Danish bovine rotavirus isolate adapted to cell culture (MA-
104), and a porcine rotavirus originating direct from faeces, both partially purified on the above mentioned immunosorbent column. Rabbits were
immunized at intervals of two weeks with an emulsion of equal amounts of
partially purified virus and Freund's incomplete adjuvant. Sera were collected before the immunization schedule started (preimmune sera), and after
subsequent immunization. All the above mentioned sera and a fetal calf
serum were tested for antibody against rotavirus using a blocking ELISA
(Askaa, 1982) using both the Danish porcine and the Danish bovine isolates
adapted to cell-culture (MA-104 cells). Only the bovine convalescent serum
and the two hyperimmune rabbit sera were found to contain anti-rotavirus
antibodies.

SDS-PAGE

Electrophoresis was performed in slab gels according to Laemmli (1970).
The separation gel (1.5 mm thick) contained 8 or 10% polyacrylamide and the
stacking gel (2 cm long) contained 4% polyacrylamide. The sample buffer
consisted of 25 mM Tris (hydroxymethyl) aminomethane (Tris), 25 mM N,N-bis
(2-hydroxymethyl) glycine (Bicine), 40% (v/v) glycerol; 4 mM trisodium
ethylenediaminetetraacetate (EDTA), 8% sodium dodecyl sulfate (SDS), 0.01%
bromophenol blue. The electrophoresis buffer consisted of Tris (6 g/l),

glycine (28.8 g/1), 0.1% SDS, pH 8.5 (King and Laemmli, 1971).

Before electrophoresis the sample buffer was added to the sample (FF or CV) and the mixture was immersed in boiling water for 3 mins or occasionally heated for 10 mins at 56°C. For comparing protein bands on the polyacrylamide gels with bands obtained on nitrocellulose sheets by the blotting technique, the gels were occasionally fixed in 25% methanol, 75% acetic acid for one hour, stained in 0.25% Coomassie blue, 50% methanol, 7.5% acetic acid for one hour 56°C and destained in 35% methanol, 7.5% acetic acid. Electrophoresis calibration kits from Pharmacia were used for molecular weight determination.

Western blotting

The separated proteins in the polyacrylamide gel were transferred electrophoretically to nitrocellulose paper (0.45 μm pore size, BIORAD). The transfer procedure has been adapted from Towbin et al. (1979), Burnette (1981) and Horzinek (personal communication, 1982) using 0.375 M Tris/HCl, pH 8.8, 20% methanol, 0.015 M SDS as transfer buffer in a Trans-Blot cell apparatus (BIO-RAD). The electrophoretic transfer was accomplished at 110 mA and 6V for 4 hours. After transfer of the proteins the molecular weight markers on the nitrocellulose sheets were stained with amido black (Towbin et al., 1979), and destained in 10% methanol, 10% acetic acid.

Immediately following transfer the residual active sites on the nitrocellulose were blocked with 2% Tween 20 for 2 mins before incubation in antiserum. This blocking procedure gives in our opinion less "background" than the saturation of additional protein binding sites with bovine serum albumin (as described by Towbin et al., 1979). The nitrocellulose sheet was incubated overnight at 4°C or 5 hours at room temperature in antisera diluted in a washing buffer consisting of 0.5 M sodium chloride, 2.7 mM potassium chloride, 1.5 mM potassium dihydrogen phosphate, 6.5 mM di-sodium hydrogen phosphate 2-hydrate, 0.05% Tween 20. After incubation in antisera, the nitrocellulose was washed three times for 10 mins in washing buffer, and incubated for 5 hours at room temperature with an anti-IgG peroxidase conjugate diluted in washing buffer. After the second incubation it was washed again three times. Occasionally the nitrocellulose was directly incubated with commercially available peroxidase-conjugated rabbit immunoglobulins to human rotavirus (Dakopatts A/S, DK). The substrate containing 250 μl orthodianisidine (stock solution 1% in methanol), 33 μl hydrogen peroxide (30%) in 100 ml 0.01 M Tris/HCl, pH 7.4 (prepared fresh) was added to the nitrocellulose sheets. After approximately 15 mins, when distinct bands had appeared, the reaction was stopped by pouring off the substrate and rinsing with distilled water. The nitrocellulose sheets were kept in water at 4°C. This procedure makes the bands appear more distinct. During the incubation the nitrocellulose sheets were placed on a rocking platform.

RESULTS

Table 1 shows the results of using different antigen preparations combined with different sera and conjugated immunoglobulins in the blotting. Five to six polypeptides with estimated molecular weight of 30K to 160K were observed.

One of the bands (68K) obtained when bovine rotavirus isolated directly from faeces was incubated with rabbit anti-bovine rotavirus (cell culture) serum originated from albumin. The same band was also obtained for the faeces without rotavirus antigen. However 5 polypeptides with estimated molecular weights of 150-160K, 140K, 60-65K, 48-51K and 30K have been identified in faeces from cattle infected with bovine rotavirus (by application of 5 samples from different farms). The 30K polypeptide was found only where the rabbit anti-porcine rotavirus (faeces) was used. Five polypeptides were also identified in faeces from swine infected with porcine rotavirus with estimated molecular weights of 150K, 145K, 99K, 62-65K and 49K (only one sample applied). A 87K large polypeptide is questionable, because a weak band was also obtained when the faecal sample without rotavirus antigen was employed. The polypeptides with estimated molecular weight of 150K and 145K were found only when the rabbit anti-bovine rotavirus (cell culture virus) was used.

When the peroxidase conjugated immunoglobulins to human rotavirus were used in the direct test, 2 polypeptides with estimated molecular weight of 49K and 30K were identified for the faecal bovine rotavirus, but only the 49K polypeptide for the faecal porcine rotavirus. No polypeptide bands were found employing the faecal samples without rotavirus antigen.

For the cell culture virus, 2 polypeptides were identified with estimated MW of 47K and 27K. The 27K polypeptide was identified only for the porcine rotavirus and only when the direct test with peroxidase conjugated immunoglobulins to human rotavirus were used. A large amount of bovine serum albumin in the cell culture preparation might be the reason for not finding the 60-65K polypeptide in these experiments. A more complete purification to get rid of the bovine serum albumin will be necessary for

TABLE 1 Results of using different antigen preparations combined with different sera.

Sera and conjugates	BOVINE FAECAL SAMPLES		PORCINE FAECAL SAMPLES		CELL CULTURE		
	pos. rotavirus antigen	neg. rotavirus antigen	pos. rotavirus antigen	neg. rotavirus antigen	bovine rotavirus infected	porcine rotavirus infected	mock infected
peroxidase conj. rabbit Ig to cow Ig	NT	NT	NT	NT	NBO	NBO	NT
peroxidase conj. swine Ig to rabbit Ig	NBO	NBO	NBO	NT	NBO	NBO	NT
* rabbit antiserum to bovine rotavirus (cell culture) 618	150-160K 140K (68K) 60-65K 48-51K	68K	150K 145K 99K (87K) 62-65K 49K	87K	NT	NT	NT
* preimmune serum 618	NBO	NBO	NBO	NT	NT	NT	NT
* rabbit antiserum to porcine rotavirus (faeces) 620	60-65K 48-51K 30K	NBO	99K (86K) 62-65K 49K	86K	47K	47K	NBO
* preimmune serum 620	NBO	NT	NBO	NT	NBO	NBO	NT
* bovine convalescent serum	NT	NT	NT	NT	47K	NT	NBO
* fetal calf serum	NT	NT	NT	NT	NBO	NT	NBO
peroxidase conj. rabbit Ig to human rotavirus	49K 30K	NBO	49K	NT	47K	47K 27K	NBO

NT = not tested
NBO = no bands obtained
* = afterwards incubated in conj. swine Ig to rabbit Ig.
* = afterwards incubated in conj. rabbit Ig. to cow Ig.

further examination of cell culture virus. No polypeptides were identified
for the mock infected cell culture.

The results reported above were obtained when the virus samples were
dissociated by immersing in boiling water for 3 mins before the SDS-PAGE.
When the virus samples were heated for 10 mins at 56°C instead, a total
dissociation of the virus proteins did not occur, and 2-3 polypeptides appeared with estimated MW of 80-85K, 95-100K and inconstantly 120K. The
band for the polypeptide with MW of 80-85K was very strong and the most intense band of all bands obtained in the experiments. No bands were obtained when samples without rotavirus antigen were treated by this method.

DISCUSSION

As seen when the results of other authors (Table 2) are compared with
the results of the present report, there is partial agreement.

TABLE 2   Comparison of the different mol. wt. values $(X10^{-3})$ of the
polypeptides reported for bovine rotavirus (this paper includes
porcine rotavirus too).

This paper	Bridger & Woode (1976)	Matsuno & Mukoyama (1979)	Novo & Esparza (1981)	Observations
160-150 145-140	125	130	102	Minor inner capsid component
99	103	115-97	91	Second most abundant component of the inner capsid
-	98	-	84	Outer capsid component
60-65	63	68	-	Outer capsid component
40-49	44	34+32.5	45	Most abundant component of the inner capsid
30	-	28	37)	Outer capsid components
-	-	24.5	34)	

Our most consistantly found polypeptide with estimated MW of 40-49K
was also the most abundantly present component in the work of Novo and
Esparza (1981) and Bridger and Woode (1976). Novo and Esparza reported it
as an inner capsid component representing 80% of total protein in single-
capsid particles. The 30K and 60-65K polypeptides are reported by Matsuno

and Mukoyama (1979) as outer capsid components. The three larger polypeptides are reported by the other authors as inner capsid components. The
strong 80-85K polypeptide band which was found when the low temperature pretreatment of the samples was used might contain the abundant 40-49K polypeptide because of the lack of this band. Some polypeptides may be lacking,
probably because of a partial loss of polypeptides from the particles during
the purification procedure. Such loss has been a problem in connection with
antiserum production in rabbits. However a low antigenicity of the polypeptides may also explain why some bands did not appear.

In our experiments, we have found it very important to use the antisera
and the anti IgG peroxidase conjugates in the optimum dilutions. If they
are used at too high concentrations, they will bind nonspecificially to the
polypeptides. Our conjugates used at a dilution of 1/500 gave no bands in
the absence of rabbit- or bovine antisera, and distinct bands after pre-
incubation in specific rabbit- or bovine antisera. Also the antigen has to
be used at its optimum dilution. The rabbit antiserum to cell culture
virus resulted in cell specific and albumin bands when cell culture virus
was used for the blotting. This indicates that more specific antisera and/
or more purified virus are needed.

REFERENCES

Askaa,J. and Bloch, B. 1981. Detection of porcine rotavirus by EM, ELISA
    and CIET. Acta Vet. Scand., 22, 32-38.
Askaa, J. 1982. Detection of antibody against porcine rotavirus in colos-
    trum and milk by a blocking ELISA test. In Current Topics in Veterin-
    ary Medicine and Animal Science, Vol. 22. "The ELISA: Enzyme-Linked
    Immunosorbent Assay in Veterinary Research and Diagnosis" (Eds.
    R.C. Wardley and J.R. Crowther). (Martinus Nijhoff, The Hague). pp.
    256-266.
Bridger, J.C. and Woode, G.N. 1976. Characterization of two particles
    types of calf rotavirus. J. Gen. Virol., 31, 245-250.
Burnette, W.N. 1981. "Western Blotting": Electrophoretic transfer of pro-
    teins from sodium dodecyl sulfate-polyacrylamide gels to unmodified
    nitrocellulose and radiographic detection with antibody and radio-
    iodinated protein A. Anal. Biochem., 112, 195-203.
Estes, M.K. and Graham, D.Y. 1980. Identification of rotaviruses of dif-
    ferent origins by the plaque-reduction test. Am. J. Vet. Res., 41,
    151-153.
Flewett, T.H., Bryden, A.S., Davies, H., Woode, G.N., Bridger, J.C. and
    Derrick, J.M. 1974. Relation between viruses from acute gastro-
    enteritis of children and newborn calves. Lancet, 2, 61-63.
Grauballe, P.C., Genner, J., Meyling, A. and Hornsleth, Å. 1977. Rapid di-
    agnosis of rotavirus infections: Comparison of electron microscopy and
    immunoelectro-osmophoresis for the detection of rotavirus in human in-
    fantile gastroenteritis. J. Gen. Virol., 35, 203-218.
Grauballe, P.C., Vestergaard, B.F., Meyling, A. and Genner, J. 1981.

144

Optimized enzyme-linked immunosorbent assay for the detection of human and bovine rotavirus in stools: Comparison with electron-microscopy, immunoelectro-osmophoresis and fluorescent antibody technique. J. Med. Virol., 7, 29-40.

King, J. and Laemmli, U.K. 1971. Polypeptides of the tail fibres of bacteriophage T4. J. Mol. Biol., 62, 465-473.

Laemmli, U.K. 1970. Cleavage of structural proteins during the assembly of the head of bacteriophage T4. Nature, 227, 680-685.

Matsuno, S. and Mukoyama, A. 1979. Polypeptides of bovine rotavirus. J. Gen. Virol., 43, 309-316.

Novo, E. and Esparza, J. 1981. Composition and topography of structural polypeptides of bovine rotavirus. J. Gen. Virol., 56, 325-335.

Shainoff, J.R. 1980. Zonal immobilisation of proteins. Biochem. Biophys. Res. Commun., 95, 690-695.

Towbin, H., Staehelin, T. and Gordon, J. 1979. Electrophoretic transfer of proteins from polyacrylamide gels to nitrocellulose sheets: Procedure and some applications. Proc. Natl. Acad. Sci. USA, 76, 4350-4354.

Woode, G.N., Bridger, J.C., Jones, J.M., Flewett, T.H., Bryden, A.S., Davies, H.A. and White, G.B.B. 1976. Morphological and antigenic relationships between viruses (rotaviruses) from acute gastroenteritis of children, calves, piglets, mice and foals. Infect. Immun., 14, 804-810.

USE OF MONOCLONAL ANTIBODIES IN VIRUS DIAGNOSIS

D. van Zaane

Central Veterinary Institute, Virology Department
Postbus 365, 8200 AJ Lelystad, The Netherlands.

INTRODUCTION

In 1975, Köhler and Milstein discovered as a spin-off result of their fundamental studies on immunoglobulin gene-expression, that lymphocytes can be immortalized by fusion with myeloma cells and thus acquire the ability to grow indefinitely and produce unlimited amounts of highly specific antibody (Köhler and Milstein, 1975). Since then, the production and application of monoclonal antibodies (MCA) has become common practice in many research areas. The enthusiasm and excitement evoked by this discovery was recently put into words by David et al. (1981) who formulated very elegantly that "the feelings experienced by an avid science fiction enthusiast watching the first astronaut plant his foot firmly on the surface of the moon could not have been dissimilar to those experienced by an immunochemist realizing the meaning of the new application of cell fusion technology presented by Köhler and Milstein".

Also in virus research, many applications have been described or are under development. However, at present large-scale use of MCA's in diagnostic assays to replace conventional antisera is not yet wide-spread. The reason for this is probably that the production, selection and characterization of MCA's with optimal and reliable properties in diagnostic assays is very time-consuming and can be hindered by many pitfalls. It is the purpose of the present overview to illustrate some of the advantages and disadvantages of the application of MCA's in virus diagnosis. However, many aspects also hold for applications in other fields. (See also reviews by Goding, 1980; Kennett et al., 1980; McMichael and Bastin, 1980; Mitchell, 1981; Oxford, 1982; Rowe, 1980; Scharff et al., 1981; Staines and Lew, 1980).

PRODUCTION

In advance, some practical aspects of MCA production seems to be worthwhile to consider. For the production of MCA's several detailed protocols have been published (e.g. Fazekas and Scheidegger, 1980; Goding, 1980; Köhler, 1980; Oi and Herzenberg, 1980).

In principle, (spleen-) lymphocytes, mostly from Balb/c mice, are fused with HAT-sensitive myeloma cells in their logarithmic growing phase, using some molecular form of polyethyleneglycol as fusing agent. In our laboratory, for each fusion an ampoule of frozen myeloma cells is thawed and cells are grown as a suspension culture in a spinner flask using RPMI 1640 medium supplemented with 15% foetal calf serum (formulation as by Fazekas and Scheidegger, 1980). Medium is added daily to maintain logarithmic growth. Thus, risks of contamination and mutation to HAT-resistance are reduced and logarithmically growing cells can very easily be harvested without damage.

It has been published that Ca^{2+} increases the toxicity of poly-ethyleneglycol for cells (Schneiderman et al., 1979). Therefore, in our procedure lymphocytes and myeloma cells are washed and fused in Ca^{2+} free medium (Eagle's minimal essential medium for suspension culture, supplemented with 0.01% w/v EDTA). After fusion, hybrid cells are selected by growth in HAT-medium, which is usually added directly after fusion or after about one day growth in non-selective medium.

Apart from an adequate fusion procedure, success in MCA production seems to be highly dependent on the protocol for immunization of the mice. In general, for production of MCA's against particulate antigens like viruses or cells, hyperimmunization followed one to two months later by one or two intravenous boosters 3-4 days before fusion appears to be adequate. However, for soluble antigens this protocol results only in a low number of positive clones. A very high yield of positive clones can be obtained by applying the immunization scheme for soluble antigens developed by Stähli et al. (1980), who injected hyperimmunized mice repeatedly with high doses of antigen during four subsequent days before fusion. Using this procedure we obtained from one spleen over 1000 independent clones producing antibody against swine IgG. The disadvantage of this immunization scheme is its length (several months), the amount of antigen required (1.5 mg for each mouse) and, in theory, the preference for low-affinity antibodies. Some of these problems might be circumvented by applying an immunization procedure described by Hudson and Hay (1980). They obtained also a high frequency of clones producing antibody against soluble antigen by injecting unprimed mice seven days before fusion with antigen in Freund's adjuvant complete followed three days later by an intravenous booster (100 μg for each injection).

APPLICATIONS

MCA's possess several advantageous properties over conventional antisera, which are in fact very heterogeneous mixtures of antibodies with
different specificity and affinity for various epitopes of (an) antigen(s).
MCA's are homogeneous reagents with specificity for one single epitope.
They can be reproducibly obtained in high titre and since hybridoma cells
can be stored in liquid nitrogen for many years, their availability is
indefinitely. Their production reduces the number of more-highly
developed experimental animals used for immunization purposes.

TABLE 1

Advantages	Disadvantages
- specificity	- laborious to produce and
- reproducibility	characterize
- high titre	- specificity might be too high
- "unlimited" availability	- instability
- reduction number of experimental	- restricted biological activity
animals	(C'-fixation, precipitation)
	- ascites tumours in mice

On the other hand, the applicability of MCA's is hindered by several
disadvantages. MCA's are laborious to produce and to characterize, their
specificity might be too high and consequently they might fail to recognize closely related variant antigens (e.g. virus strains). In addition,
they can be instable to alterations in physical conditions or to storage,
they display a restricted biological activity (e.g. C'-fixation, cytotoxi-
city, precipitation) and finally, MCA-producing cells have to be grown as
ascites tumours in mice to produce samples with high titre in an easy way
(Table 1). Thus, several problems can be met in applying MCA's.
Some of these and a possible solution are summarized in Table II.

Nevertheless, MCA's can be very useful and sometimes essential in
viral diagnosis (Table III). They are the reagents of choice for an inter-
national standardization of diagnostic techniques, for the identification
and fine-typing of closely related viruses or strains, for antigen purification via immuno-adsorbens columns or directly in solid-phase assays, and
when high amounts of specific antibody are required.

TABLE II

Problems	Solution
- too high specificity	- mixture of MCA's
- restricted biological activity	- selection of mouse-isotype; mixture
- low affinity	- selection for high-affinity MCA
- cross-reactivity	- other MCA
- competition between MCA's	- use of MCA's to different epitopes

In future, MCA's against idiotype determinants, which mimic the antigenic determinant inducing that particular idiotype of antibody, might replace antigen in diagnostic assays (e.g. serological assays or competitive assays for antigen detection) and in this way circumventing laborious purification procedures. However, synthetic polypeptides, if available, might be more appropriate for this purpose.

TABLE III

Applications in veterinary diagnosis
- standardization
- identification
- fine-typing
- antigen purification
- anti-idiotype reagents
- high amount of specific antibody

Several of the applications of MCA's and related problems will be illustrated below.

Specificity versus too high specificity

Hog cholera or classical swine fever is a wide-spread economically important disease of swine. The diagnosis, mainly based on immunofluorescence on frozen sections of tonsils of suspected animals, is severely hindered by the cross-reaction between swine fever virus (SFV) and bovine viral diarrhoea virus (BVDV). The latter virus can also infect pigs. In addition, antibodies to BVDV in swine sera cause false-positive results in serological surveys for SFV-antibody, unless a time-consuming and

laborious neutralization test is employed. In our institute, two MCA
producing clones were obtained which neutralize SFV strain Brescia but
are unreactive with BVDV (Table IV). So, these reagents are candidates

TABLE IV

MCA's to swine fever virus (C. Terpstra, pers. comm.)		
Neutralization	clone 21.1	clone 21.2
SFV Brescia	++	+
BVD Oregon C24	-	-

to be used for the differential diagnosis of SFV and BVDV infections.
However, these reagents seems to be too specific since they did not
recognize some SFV strains using an indirect immunofluorescence test
(Table V) (Dr. C. Terpstra, pers. comm.). The production of other MCA's
with a broader specificity for variant SFV strains or the use of mixtures
of MCA's can circumvent this problem.

TABLE V

MCA's to swine fever virus (C. Terpstra)		
IIF	clone 21.1	clone 21.2
SFV strains:		
Henken	-	-
V.d.Bergen	+	+
331	--	+
Brescia	+	+
Bai	-	+
BVD strains:		
NADL	-	-
1138	-	-
Oregon C24	-	-

MCA's have been applied for the identification and fine-typing of
several other viruses (e.g. influenza, rabies, New Castle disease virus,
foot-and-mouth disease virus, herpes simplex virus, cytomegalovirus. See

Gerhard et al., 1981; Phillips et al., 1982; Koprowski et al., 1980;
Russell et al., 1983; McCullough et al., 1982; Peterson et al., 1983;
Nilheden et al., 1983; Goldstein et al., 1982).

In case of HSV, type 1 and 2 could be distinguished with MCA's as
faithfully as with restriction enzyme analysis (Peterson et al., 1983),
whereas application of conventional antisera yielded 34% intermediate
classifications. In another type of assay, using an immunoperoxidase
technique, one single plaque of HSV type 1 could be identified among 200
HSV type 2 plaques (Nilheden et al., 1983).

Specificity versus cross-reactivity

Although MCA's react with one single antigenic determinant of a particular antigen, they can react with unrelated antigens, possessing the
same or a very similar determinant. In contrast to conventional antisera,
MCA's cannot be absorbed with the cross-reacting antigen.

For our studies on the mucosal immune system in cattle, the availability of monospecific reagents for bovine Ig-isotypes G_1, G_2, M and A is
essential. In our hands, conventional immuno-absorbed antisera appeared to
be highly cross-reactive in a very sensitive Elisa assay (Fig. 1). Therefore, we produced MCA's against the bovine Ig-isotypes. Several MCA's were
obtained which were specific for IgG, IgG_1, IgG_2 and IgA. However, MCA's
against IgM crossreacted partially with IgA (Fig. 1). Further experiments
excluded that this cross-reactivity was due to a contamination of the IgA
preparation with IgM (Van Zaane and IJzerman, manuscript in preparation).
In this case, the cross-reactivity was not so surprising since IgM and
IgA are related molecules. However, cross-reactivity of MCA's was also
observed for SV40 T-antigen and a normal host cell component, for Thy-1
and V_k, and for a glycoprotein of HSV and glycolipid of host cells (Ref.
in Lane and Koprowski, 1982).

In our study on the mucosal immune system of calves, MCA's against
bovine Ig-isotypes were successfully applied in class-specific Elisa's
for the detection of antibodies against rotavirus in serum and faeces
(Van Zaane and IJzerman, manuscript in preparation).

Specificity, standardization, unlimited availability versus competition

An eradication programme for avian leukosis virus (ALV) in commercial
flocks was developed by Rispens et al. (1976) and is based on the detection
and culling of laying hens which transmit ALV via their eggs to their off-

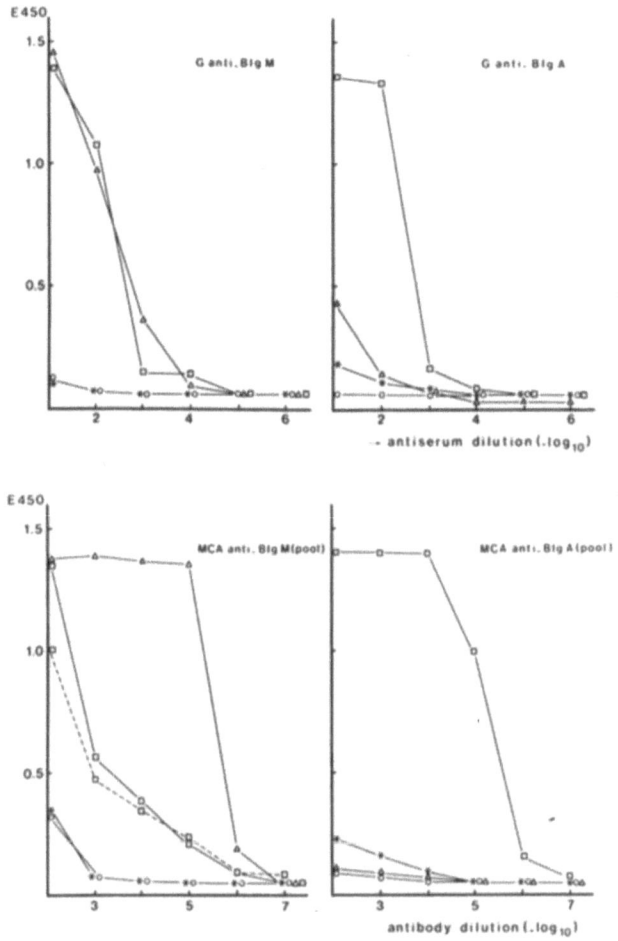

Fig. 1 Specificity of conventional antisera (upper panels) and
monoclonal antibodies (lower panels) against bovine IgM or IgA
in an indirect Elisa. Sequential ten-fold dilutions of antibody
preparations indicated in the figure were tested in Elisa-plates
coated with purified IgG_1 (*), IgG_2 (o), IgM (△), IgA (□) or
affinity purified IgA (---□---). Binding was monitored by a horse
radish peroxidase conjugated second antibody. The purified Ig-
preparations were gifts of Dr. B.A. Bokhout, Central Veterinary
Institute, Lelystad, The Netherlands.

spring. Detection of virus containing eggs by virusisolation, as used
during the experimental development of the programme, is not suited for
large scale application in practice. Therefore, a double antibody sandwich
(DAS) Elisa was developed for the detection of gs-antigen of ALV in eggs
(G.F. de Boer, unpublished results). Conventional antisera produced in
rabbits by injecting purified ALV react with normal chicken components
and had to be absorbed. Hamsters bearing Rous sarcoma virus induced
tumours (expressing gs-antigen) yielded only low amounts of specific antisera. Again, MCA's as catching and/or conjugated antibody seemed to be the
reagents of choice. However, MCA's from clone 8A and 8B appeared to differ
in their ability to function as catching antibody in the DAS-Elisa. (Table
VI) (Dr. G.F. de Boer and A.D.M.E. Osterhaus, pers. comm.). This can be
explained by differences in affinity, physico-chemical properties or in

TABLE VI

DAS-Elisa for ALV gs-antigen			sensitivity*
1) R anti-AMV	- testsample -	HA anti-GS-HRP	1/1024
2) MCA 8A (anti-P27)	- testsample -	HA anti-GS-HRP	1/1024
3) MCA 8B (anti-P27)	- testsample -	HA anti-GS-HRP	1/256
4) MCA 8A (anti-P27)	- testsample -	MCA 8B (anti-P27)-HRP	neg
5) MCA 8A (anti-P27A)	- testsample -	MCA anti-P27B-HRP	?

*endpoint dilution of gs^+ embryo testsample

exposure of antigen binding sites. It has been shown by David et al.
(1981) that MCA's with good and equal properties as conjugated antibodies
display very different properties as catching antibody. When MCA's 8A and
8B were used as catching and conjugated antibody, respectively, in one
assay, a completely negative result was obtained, which indicates that
MCA's 8A and 8B are directed against the same epitope of the gs-antigen
or against epitopes which are very close to each other.

The use of MCA's that recognize distinct epitopes of the same antigen
or different antigens of the same virus can result in highly specific
assays. In this way, Goodall et al. (1981) developed a sensitive assay
for the detection of hepatitis B antigen in serum or plasma. In some
cases, conventional antisera still seem to be preferable (e.g. detection
of Toxoplasma gondii; Aranjo et al., 1980) and result in more sensitive
assays (detection of influenza virus by a double antibody sandwich

immunofluometric assay; Phillips et al., 1982).

Antigen purification

Purified preparations of virus antigens are often used in assays for the detection of anti-viral antibody. With the use of MCA's to a (particular) virus (antigen) large immunoadsorbens columns can be prepared to achieve a rapid and simple purification procedure. Even more simple is the purification of virus (antigen) from crude samples by direct binding to a MCA coated solid phase. Thus, it appears to be possible to bind gs-antigen of maedi-visna virus directly from tissue culture medium to an Elisa-plate coated with MCA against maedi-visna virus. However, the use of these plates in serological diagnosis for maedi-visna virus antibody has been unsuccessful until now (D.J. Houwers and J. Schaake, pers. comm.).

Recently Portetelle et al. (1983) reported a similar and successful assay for the detection of antibody against bovine leukosis virus glycoprotein gp51. They selected a catching MCA which allowed the binding of gp51 in such a way that epitopes of gp51 recognized in vivo were optimally exposed. This work is the subject of the next paper.

Single incubation step test, cooperative and stick-Elisa

Since non-competitive MCA reagents can be selected for application in DAS-assays for (viral) antigen detection, it has become possible to incubate a test sample and a labelled MCA simultaneously with a MCA coated solid phase. Based on this principle a rapid and very sensitive assay for the detection of hepatitis B antigen (Goodall et al., 1982) and α-foetoprotein (Uotila et al., 1981) was developed (detection limit 0,5 ng/ml and 1.0 ng/ml, respectively).

This also means that stick-Elisa's can be developed: MCA against a pathogen are coated on plastic sticks and the conjugated second MCA is absorbed in a reversible way. When the assay stick is put into the test sample, the conjugated MCA will solubilize and subsequently bind to the antigen if present. The antigen or the immuno-complex can bind to the MCA coated stick. After washing, the stick has to be incubated in a solution of substrate of which the product precipitates on the solid phase. When MCA's for different viruses or strains are coated on different areas of a stick, even differential diagnosis or fine-typing should be possible.

154

Recently, a cooperative assay for antigen detection was described
(Ehrlich and Moyle, 1983). It is based on the formation of circular soluble complexes of antigen and two non-competitive monoclonals resulting in
a higher binding affinity for the antigen than that of each individual
MCA. This non-competitive assay is highly specific and sensitive and might
be useful for the direct detection of viral antigens in test samples without virus isolation.

CONCLUSIONS

The application of MCA's in virus diagnosis seems to be very promising but is also full of pitfalls. Therefore, extreme care should be taken
before a diagnostic test based on MCA is developed and distributed for in
practice use.

Finally, one should consider that the use of highly specific MCA's
for the diagnosis of pathogens may result in the escape of variant strains
not recognized by a particular MCA. Thus, MCA's could exert evolutionary
pressure towards the survival of "new" pathogens (David et al., 1981).

ACKNOWLEDGEMENTS

I am very grateful to Dr. C. Terpstra, Dr. G.F. de Boer,
Dr. A.D.M.E. Osterhaus, Dr. D.J. Houwers, Mr. J. IJzerman and Mr.
J. Schaake for allowing me to refer to their recent unpublished results.

REFERENCES

Aranjo, F.G., Handman, E. and Remington, J.S. 1980. Use of monoclonal
antibodies to detect antigens of Toxoplasma gondii in serum and
other body fluids. Infect. Immun., 30, 12-16.
David, G.S., Present, W., Mirtinis, J., Wang, R., Bartolomew, R., Desmond,
W. and Sevier, E.D. 1981. Monoclonal antibodies in the detection of
hepatitis infection. Med. Lab. Sci., 38, 341-348.
Ehrlich, P.H. and Moyle, W.R. 1983. Co-operative immunoassays: Ultra-
sensitive assays with mixed monoclonal antibodies. Science, 221,
279-281.
Fazekas de St. Groth, S. and Scheidegger, D. 1980. Production of monoclonal
antibodies: Strategy and tactics. J. Immunol. Meth., 35, 1-21.
Gerhard, W., Yewdell, J., Frankel, M.E. and Webster, R. 1981. Antigenic
structure of influenza virus haemagglutinin defined by hybridoma
antibodies. Nature (London), 290, 713-717.
Goding, J.W. 1980. Antibody production by hybridomas. J. Immunol. Meth.,
39, 285-308.
Goldstein, L.C., McDougall, J., Hackman, R., Meyers, J.D., Thomas, E.D.
and Nowinski, R.C. 1982. Monoclonal antibodies to cytomegalovirus:
rapid identification of clinical isolates and preliminary use in
diagnosis of cytomegalovirus pneumonia. Infect. Immun., 38, 273-281.

Goodall, A.H., Meek, F.L., Waters, J.A., Miescher, G.C., Janossy, G. and
Thomas, H.C. 1982. A rapid one-step radiometric assay for hepatitis
B surface antigen utilising monoclonal antibodies. J. Immun. Meth.,
52, 167-174.

Goodall, A.H., Miescher, G., Meek, F.M., Janossy, G. and Thomas, H.C. 1981.
Monoclonal antibodies in a solid-phase radiometric assay for HBsAg.
Med. Lab. Sci., 38, 349-354.

Hudson, L. and Hay, F.C. 1980. Practical Immunology, 2nd edition
(Blackwell Scientific Publication, Oxford).

Kennett, R.H., McKearn, T.J. and Bechtol, K.B. 1980. Monoclonal antibodies (Plenum Press, New York).

Köhler, G. 1980. Hybridoma techniques (Cold Spring Harbor Laboratory
Manual, Cold Spring Harbor).

Köhler, G. and Milstein, C. 1975. Continuous cultures of fused cells
secreting antibody of predefined specificity. Nature (London), 256,
495-497.

Koprowski, H. and Wiktor, T. 1980. Monoclonal antibodies against rabies
virus. In Monoclonal Antibodies (Ed. R.H. Kennett, T.J. McKearn and
K.B. Bechtol) (Plenum Press, New York). pp. 335-351.

Lane, D. and Koprowski, H. 1982. Molecular recognition and the future
of monoclonal antibodies. Nature (London), 296, 200-202.

McCullough, K.C. and Butcher, R. 1982. Monoclonal antibodies against foot-
and-mouth disease virus 146S and 12S particles. Arch. Virol., 74,
1-9.

McMichael, A.J. and Bastin, J.M. 1980. Clinical applications of monoclonal
antibodies. Immunology Today, 1, 56-61.

Mitchell, G.F. 1981. Hybridoma antibodies in immunodiagnosis of parasitic
infection. Immunology Today, 2, 140-142.

Nilheden, E., Jeansson, S. and Vahlne, A. 1983. Typing of herpes simplex
virus by an enzyme-linked immunosorbent assay with monoclonal antibodies. J. Clin. Microbiol., 17, 677-680.

Oi, V.T. and Herzenberg, L.A. 1980. Immunoglobulin-producing hybrid cell
lines. In Selected Methodes in cellular Immunology (Eds. B.B. Mishell
and S.M. Shiigi) (W.H. Freeman and Co, San Fransisco).

Oxford, J. 1982. The use of monoclonal antibodies in virology. J. Hyg.
Camb., 88, 361-368.

Peterson, E., Schmidt, O.W., Goldstein, L.C., Nowinski, R.C. and Corey, L.
1983. Typing of clinical herpes simplex virus isolates with mouse
monoclonal antibodies to herpes simplex virus type 1 and 2:
comparison with type-specific rabbit antisera and restriction endonuclease analysis of viral DNA. J. Clin. Microbiol., 17, 92-96.

Phillips, D.J., Galland, G.G., Reimer, C.B. and Kendal, A.P. 1982.
Evaluation of a solid-phase immunoassay with fluorescein isothio-
cyanate-conjugated heterogeneous or monoclonal antibodies for
identification of virus isolates, with influenza virus as a model.
J. Clin. Microbiol., 15, 931-937.

Portetelle, D., Bruck, C., Mammerickx, M. and Burny, A. 1983. Use of monoclonal antibody in an Elisa test for the detection of antibodies to
bovine leukemia virus. J. Vir. Meth., 6, 19-29.

Rispens, B.H., De Boer, G.F., Hoogerbrugge, A. and Van Vloten, J. 1976.
A method for the control of lymphoid leukosis in chickens. J. Nat.
Cancer Inst., 57, 1151-1156.

Rowe, D.S. 1980. The role of monoclonal antibody technology in immuno-
parasitology. Immunology Today, 1, 30-33.

Russell, P.H. and Alexander, D.J. 1983. Antigenic variation of Newcastle
disease virus strains detected by monoclonal antibodies. Arch. Virol.,

75, 243-253.

Scharff, M.D., Roberts, S. and Thamanna, P. 1981. Monoclonal antibodies. J. Inf. Dis., 143, 346-351.

Schneiderman, S., Farber, J.L. and Baserga, R. 1979. A simple method for decreasing the toxicity of polyethyleneglycol in mammalian cell hybridization. Somat. Cell Genet., 5, 263-269.

Stähli, C., Staehelin, T., Miggiano, V., Schmidt, J. and Häring, P. 1980. High frequencies of antigen-specific hybridomas: dependence on immunization parameters and prediction by spleen cell analysis. J. Immunol. Meth., 32, 297-304.

Staines, N.A. and Lew, A.M. 1980. Whither monoclonal antibodies? Immunology, 40, 287-293.

Uotila, M., Ruoslahti, E. and Engvall, E. 1981. Two-site sandwich enzyme immunoassay with monoclonal antibodies to human alpha-fetoprotein. J. Immunol. Meth., 42, 11-15.

BOVINE LEUKOSIS - RECENT DEVELOPMENTS WITH USE
OF MONOCLONAL ANTIBODIES AND ELISA TESTS

D. Portetelle[1,2], C. Bruck[1], M. Mammerickx[3] and A. Burny[1,2]

1. Department of Molecular Biology, University of Brussels,
1640 Rhode-St-Genese.
2. Faculty of Agronomy, 5800 Gembloux.
3. National Institute for Veterinary Research, 1180 Uccle,
Belgium.

ABSTRACT

A variant of the enzyme-linked immunosorbent assay (ELISA) technique involving the use of a specially selected monoclonal antibody against the BLV envelope glycoprotein gp51 yields a highly sensitive, practical and cheap method for the detection of Bovine Leukemia virus (BLV) antibodies, gp51 antigen and for the measurement of antigenic variations in the gp51 molecule.

INTRODUCTION

The enzootic form of bovine leukosis, a contagious, typical herd disease, is induced by bovine leukemia virus (BLV), a retrovirus which is exogenous to the bovine species.

Serological surveys of the cattle population seem to be the only approach for the early detection of BLV infection and the adequate basis for an efficient policy of eradication of the disease. Because the antibodies against the envelope glycoprotein BLV gp51 appear earlier after experimental infection and their titre is consistently higher than the antibodies against the internal protein p24, a test involving the gp51 antigen is the most sensitive method for the early detection of BLV infection (for review, see Burny et al., 1980).

In our laboratory, liquid phase radioimmunoassay (LPRIA) involving iodinated gp51 has repeatedly been shown to be the most sensitive test (Mammerickx et al., 1980; Portetelle et al., 1980). An optimised agar gel immunodiffusion test involving gp51 and other BLV proteins shows good agreement with LPRIA, detects anti-BLV antibodies soon after seroconversion and is moreover efficient for eradication of bovine leucosis (Mammerickx et al., 1978).

The recent development of enzyme immunoassays has elicited great interest among scientists concerned with the seroepidemiology of bovine leukosis, but so far, results have been disappointing. (Hoff-Jorgensen, 1980; Ressang et al., 1980; Manz et al.,1981; Altaner et al., 1982; Graves et al., 1982; Maris et al., 1983).

The basic principles of enzyme immunoassays are similar to those developed for quantitative radioimmunoassays but the measurement of the enzyme activity replaces the counting of radioactivity (De Savingny et al., 1980). The heterogeneous enzyme immunoassays, popularly named ELISA (enzyme-linked immunosorbent assay), take advantage of a solid phase to separate the free enzyme-labelled antigen or antibody from the specific antigen-antibody complexes containing the enzyme-labelled antigen or antibody. Enzyme immunoassays which do not imply the use of a solid phase are based on antibody-mediated changes in enzyme activity. This procedure is defined as a homogeneous enzyme immunoassay. At present, only ELISA appears to be applicable in viral diagnosis   (Avrameas, 1983).

An efficient ELISA procedure implies a high degree of specific binding versus a low degree of non-specific binding to the solid phase used. These performance characteristics are dependent to a great extent on the binding characteristics and the purity of immunoreactants involved. The availability of immunoglobulin preparations with every molecule directed against an antigen of choice should improve the kinetics of the antigen-antibody reaction and thus the sensitivity and the specificity of immunoassays.

For this reason, investigators concerned with immunoassay systems are particularly interested in the evolving technology related to the production and development of monoclonal antibodies (Yolken, 1983). The potential advantages of monoclonal antibodies for immunoassay systems are numerous and are summarised elsewhere (Van Zaane, this book; Langone and Van Vunakis, 1983).

Although monoclonal antibodies can be utilised in a wide variety of immunoassays including radioimmunoassays and immunofluorescent assays, our work has focused on adapting monoclonal antibodies to the ELISA technology in BLV research.

The principle of the use of ELISA test is largely accepted in veterinary laboratories since these assays use stable and non-radioactive reagents. This stability can also take maximal advantage of the high consistency offered by the homogeneous and monospecific nature of monoclonal antibodies.

PRINCIPLE OF THE METHOD

For this study, a variant of the classical ELISA technique is described, which involves the use of a gp51-specific monoclonal antibody. From a panel of 15 monoclonal antibodies directed against gp51, the antibody providing maximal exposure of gp51 antigenic sites recognised by bovine antisera was selected. This specially selected purified anti-gp51 monoclonal antibody is adsorbed to the wells of a microtitre plate to which it specifically binds the antigen contained in a non-purified BLV preparation.

Bovine antibodies reacting then with gp51 can be detected by an enzyme-coupled antibovine immunoglobulin immunoreactant. If we use monoclonal antibodies directed against the different independent epitopes on the gp51 molecule as anti-gp51-peroxidase conjugate, we can search for BLV gp51 or BLV particles in complex media. If we first adsorb each of the monoclonal antibodies on the solid-phase, select for the gp51 in a non-purified preparation and then reveal the presence of gp51 with a mixture of the different monoclonal antibodies conjugated to the peroxidase, we can define antigenic variations in different BLV isolates (Fig. 1).

IMPORTANT TECHNICAL CONSIDERATIONS

Our ELISA tests use an antibody immobilised on a solid-phase. Finally, the enzyme-labelled antibodies react with the specific antibody-antigen complex but also in a non-specific way with eventual antigenic structures adsorbed to the solid phase.

The specificity, the sensitivity and the reproducibility of the ELISA tests depend on several factors: the solid phase, the monoclonal antibody, the purity of this preparation, the antigen preparation, the saturation protein, dilutions of serum used, incubation time and temperature, reaction volumes, non-ionic detergent, properties of the enzyme-antibody conjugate, enzyme substrate.

1. Choice of the monoclonal antibody:

The production of monoclonal anti-gp51 antibodies has been described previously (Bruck et al., 1982 a, b). Monoclonal reagents used in this study were purified from mouse ascitic fluids by DEAE-Affigel blue (BIORAD) chromatography (Bruck et al., 1982c) and stored in aliquots at -80°C.

The monoclonal reagent used to bind gp51 was chosen from a panel of 15 monoclonal antibodies directed against 8 independent epitopes on the gp51 molecule.

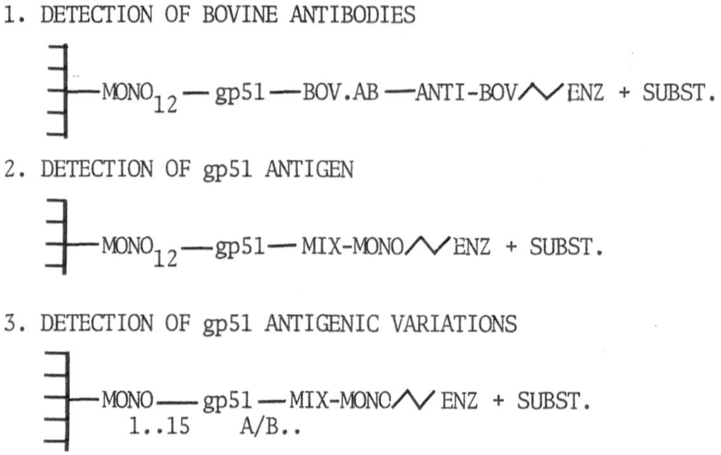

1. DETECTION OF BOVINE ANTIBODIES

$\dashv$ —MONO$_{12}$ — gp51 — BOV.AB — ANTI-BOV $\diagdown\diagup$ ENZ + SUBST.

2. DETECTION OF gp51 ANTIGEN

$\dashv$ —MONO$_{12}$ — gp51 — MIX-MONO $\diagdown\diagup$ ENZ + SUBST.

3. DETECTION OF gp51 ANTIGENIC VARIATIONS

$\dashv$ —MONO —— gp51 — MIX-MONO $\diagdown\diagup$ ENZ + SUBST.
     1..15   A/B..

MONO	:	Monoclonal antibody.
1...12	:	Number.
BOV.AB	:	Bovine antibodies.
MIX	:	Mixture of monoclonal antibodies.
A/B	:	Different BLV isolates.
ANTI-BOV:		Antibovine immunoglobulins.
ENZ	:	Enzyme (peroxidase or β-galactosidase).
SUBST	:	Enzyme substrate.

Fig. 1   Schematic representation of the ELISA tests.

Since the anti-gp51 antibodies produced by infected cattle were shown
to be directed mainly against a limited region on gp51 (Portetelle et al.,
1980) and more precisely sites, F,G,H defined with monoclonal antibodies
(Bruck et al., 1983), the choice of the monoclonal antibody to bind gp51
to the solid phase was based upon obtaining optimal exposure of the relevant antigenic sites F,G,H to the bovine antibodies. This was determined
in a sandwich solid phase radioimmunoassay as below:

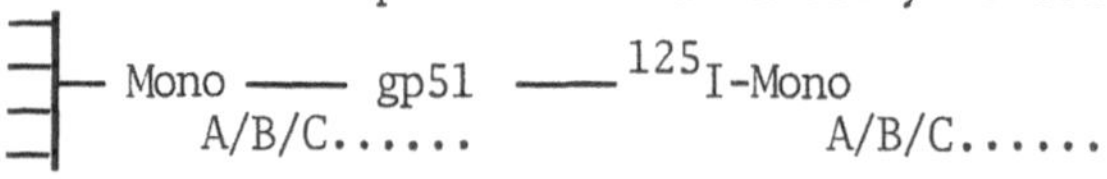

$\dashv$ — Mono —— gp51 —— ^{125}I-Mono
    A/B/C......   A/B/C......

With the monoclonal antibody GA12 directed against site E, the optimal
exposure of the bound antigen was obtained for the binding of monoclonal
antibodies against sites F,G,H and thus for the binding of bovine natural
antibodies. Minimal non-specific binding and minimal background were also
observed with this monoclonal antibody (Portetelle et al., 1983b).

2. Choice of the purification method for monoclonal antibodies:

The use of DEAE-Affigel Blue chromatography for the purification of monoclonal antibodies from ascitic fluids (Bruck et al., 1982a) leads to minimal non-specific binding in our ELISA tests (Portetelle et al., 1983b) probably because proteins involved in non-specific binding are retained on the column. It is thus important to use the purest antibody preparations available to coat the plastic surface.

3. Choice of the microtitre plate:

Microtitre plates specially treated to increase their fixation capacity (for use in enzyme immunoassay) are not suitable in our ELISA system for the detection of bovine antibodies to BLV with an excess of enzyme-labelled anti-immunoglobulin reagent. High background values and high non-specific binding were observed with these plates: we use normal microtitre plates to ensure optimal specificity (Portetelle et al., 1983b).

However, the treated plates are suitable for the detection of gp51 antigen or gp51 antigenic variations because maximal absorption of the monoclonal antibody to the well provides maximal sensitivity of these tests.

4. Choice of an inert protein:

To minimise non-specific binding and background, sites on the solid-phase are saturated with an inert protein. We have tested several sources of inert protein: bovine serum albumin (BSA), gelatin and serum from different animal species. In our system, only BSA (Sigma A9647 or other commercial BSA with equivalent quality) seems to give satisfactory results. Fraction V of BSA from certain preparations may contain contaminants which cross-react with bovine immunoglobulins and the conjugate. With other proteins, high cross-reactivity with the anti-bovine immunoglobulin conjugate is observed (gelatin contains fragments of bovine immunoglobulins).

5. Properties of the enzyme-protein conjugate:

Conjugate effectiveness depends on both the enzyme and the antibody used, and also on the conjugation procedure chosen to link the two, and plays a very important role in the development of ELISA tests. This is especially true for the detection of bovine antibodies to BLV. However, in the case of gp51 detection with the monoclonal antibodies mixture labelled with peroxidase, no special problem exists, probably because of the purity and the homogeneity of the monoclonal antibody preparations.

5.1 Enzymes:

We use only two enzymes in our system: horseradish peroxidase and E. coli β-galactosidase. These enzymes possess a high substrate turnover number, do not lose much of their activity after linkage to the antibody and remain stable at room temperature throughout the periods usually required for ELISA assays. In commercial preparations, the highest specific activity (and thus purity) is generally observed with peroxidase. However, β-galactosidase is known to give the lowest non-specific binding (Avrameas, 1983).

5.2 Coupling procedures:

Antibodies (Ab) are coupled by the periodate-oxidation method to the peroxidase (POD) preparation in a molar ratio POD: Ab = 2.5:1 (Portetelle et al., 1983a). The SH groups of β-galactosidase (GAL) can be linked to Fab fragments with a thiol-reacting agent (molar ratio 1:1) (O'Sullivan and Marks, 1981).

These coupling procedures produce a homogeneous population of conjugates which are able to detect the presence of bovine antibodies with the maximum of sensitivity. It has been reported that a higher molecular ratio in the conjugates increases the sensitivity but also increases non-specific reactions (O'Sullivan et al., 1981).

5.3 Choice of the anti-bovine immunoglobulins antibodies:

So far, we have tested three different anti-bovine antibodies conjugates for their capacity to yield the minimal non-specific binding in the detection of specific bovine antibodies.
1. Fab fragments from goat anti-bovine immunoglobulins - POD.
2. Fab fragments from goat anti-bovine immunoglobulins - GAL.
3. Fab fragments from rabbit anti-goat immunoglobulins - POD.

All of these Fab preparations are purified by affinity chromatography on bovine immunoglobulins immobilised on AH-Sepharose (Portetelle et al., 1983a).

We have tested conjugates (1) and (2) on a large scale (Mammerickx et al., 1983), the best results were observed with the β-galactosidase conjugate. Conjugate (3) seems as promising as the β-galactosidase conjugate (unpublished observations).

Protein A from Staphylococcus aureus appears to be a poor reagent for detecting specific bovine antibodies, as it possesses a very low affinity for bovine immunoglobulins.

Conjugates based on the biotin-streptavidin or avidin interaction yielded a higher amplification of the specific signal but a simultaneous increase of the non-specific signal.

5.4 Choice of the enzyme substrate:

Several different chromogenic and fluorogenic substrates are available (Avrameas, 1983). β-galactosidase activity can be easily determined with 0-nitrophenyl-B-D-galactose, using a spectrophotometer at 410 nm.

In the case of peroxidase, several chromogenic donors have been used for their spectrophotometric measurement. The first results were obtained with 0-phenylenediamine, a substance that gives highly sensitive and reliable measurements at 492 nm (Portetelle et al., 1983a; Mammerickx et al., 1983). Other highly sensitive marker substances, like ABTS, 0-dianisidine and tetramethylbenzidine are also available. Tetramethylbenzidine appears to give a high specific signal versus a low non-specific signal and is a non-hazardous substance (Table 1). Chloro-1-naphthol,

TABLE 1   Effect of the peroxidase substrate on the specificity of the BLV ELISA test for the detection of specific bovine antibodies.

Substrate	Index value
O-Phenylenediamine	100
O-Dianisidine	118
Tetramethylbenzidine	158

Conjugate   : Fab fragments from rabbit antigoat Ig-POD.
Serum dilution tested : 1/200.
Index value   : Specific OD for reference positive serum
                        divided by specific OD of reference negative
                        serum.
Data are expressed as percentage of the minimal index value observed.

diaminobenzidine, diethylcarbazole yield poor sensitivity in the detection of POD activity. Chromogenic substrates with spontaneous oxidation should be avoided (brown colour of O-phenylenedianine).

6. Determination of the optimal reaction conditions
6.1 Binding of monoclonal antibody:

The quantity of antibody fixed to the solid-phase is of critical importance in the establishment of an efficient ELISA test. Coating at high antibody concentration (300 ng per well) enhances the specific binding of gp51 antigen in the case of gp51 detection (law of mass action) and thus the sensitivity. A dose of 100 ng monoclonal antibody per well is optimal for the detection of bovine antibodies to BLV (Portetelle et al., 1983a); if 300 ng are added, more gp51 is involved in the titration test and the sensitivity is reduced. The use of less than 100 ng of monoclonal antibody increases the sensitivity of the test but requires longer incubation of the antigen - bovine antibody reaction and also increases the risk of non-specific binding with some bovine sera.

6.2 Binding of gp51 antigen:

Precoated plates (monoclonal antibody - gp51) for the detection of bovine antibodies to BLV can be prepared in advance and stored (at 4°C for at least one month). Four day culture supernatant of a BLV-infected fetal lamb kidney cell line (FLK) (Van Der Maaten et al., 1976) is used as a source of antigen. The culture medium is MEM supplied with non-essential amino-acids, kanamycin and 10% heat inactivated fetal calf serum. Minimal non-specific binding and background are observed with fetal calf serum versus newborn calf serum.

Cell debris are eliminated by centrifugation and filtration (0.45 μ); 50 μl of supernatant (more than 10 ng gp51) is mixed with 50 μl saturation buffer (2% bovine serum albumin in a high phosphate - 0.2M - concentration buffer to minimise pH variation) and incubated for a minimum time of 24 h. This relatively long incubation time necessary for maximal yield of the system is required because of the low antigen concentration used and the low avidity of monoclonal antibody GA12 for gp51 (Bruck et al., 1982a). For the detection of gp51, a maximum volume of 200 μl containing the saturation buffer and the non-ionic detergent Tween 80 (maximum 2%) is generally used and incubated 16 h at 4°C.

6.3 Influence of reaction volume, detergent, time and temperature:
We have repeatedly shown that incubation at room temperature or 37°C

appears to be deleterious to the gp51 antibody reaction (Portetelle et al., 1980; 1983a). Reaction of antibody with gp51 is more complete when the incubation temperature is 4°C. A standard incubation time of 4 h is generally used for the conjugates. Monoclonal antibody is generally coated in a 50 µl volume. Incubation of the bovine serum dilution in 200 µl slightly decreases the sensitivity of the detection test (16 h as standard incubation time), but most interestingly also the non-specific adsorption of negative BLV serum: non-specific immunoglobulin bound to the upper part of the well is not revealed by addition of 50 µl of conjugate.

Non-specific adsorption can be reduced but not excluded by including a non-ionic detergent in the medium during the incubation (2% for bovine serum) and washing steps (0.2%). We have used Tween 80, either alone (0.2% in conjugate dilution) or supplemented with BSA (2%) in other cases (see Appendix).

6.4 Influence of serum dilution:

The quantity of bovine antibodies fixed to the solid phase is of critical importance in the establishment of an efficient ELISA test. High concentrations of bovine antibody reduce specific binding and enhance non-specific binding (steric hindrance). When the dilution of bovine serum used is too low, the specific binding on the solid phase will be small and consequently the sensitivity will be reduced. It is important to find the optimal dilution for the ELISA system under investigation.

Sera from a known infected herd and from nineteen BLV-free herds were tested at four dilutions: 1/20, 1/60, 1/180, 1/540 at the same time with the β-galactosidase conjugate (2) (Mammerickx et al., 1983). The optical density was read and the animals are classified according to the optical density scored. The best results were observed with the dilution 1/60. At this dilution the two cattle populations were the most distinctly separated. The mean value of optical density (OD) observed with positive animals was in the range of 0.500-0.750 OD; the mean OD value for negative animals was in the range o.001-0.025 OD. A suitable cut-off value between the two cattle populations appeared to be situated at the optical density 0.150 for the serum dilution 1/60.

ADVANTAGES

We have found that specially selected monoclonal antibodies can be

used to obtain sensitive immunoassay systems. The main limitation of monoclonal antibody technology in immunoassays continues to be the tediousness
of the procedures necessary for generation and selection of the hybridoma
clones (Langone and Van Vunakis, 1983).

The system so designed for BLV research was shown to be as sensitive
as gp51 LPRIA for the detection of bovine antibodies (Portetelle et al.,
1983a); 10 pg gp51 per well can also be detected with our ELISA system
although our classical radioimmunoassay can detect 50 pg. This difference
is due to the stability and the homogeneity of the immunoreactants in the
ELISA test and the accelerated radiolysis observed with gp51 if specific
activity is higher than $2X10^6$ dpm/µg. The sensitivity of this system takes
advantage of the increased concentration of specific antibody on the solid-
phase offered by monoclonal antibodies (Table 2), and the increased range
of antigen-binding sites offered by the polyclonal antibodies or the
mixture of monoclonal antibodies as conjugates.

TABLE 2   Concentration of specific antibody in different
           preparations.

Antibody preparation	Concentration of specific antibody (%)
Monoclonal	100
Affinity purified	30[*]
Hyperimmune	10[*]

(*) Relative concentration, in comparison with the mono-
    clonal antibody preparation.

Sensitivity and specificity are assured by the fact that the use of
a monoclonal antibody rather than a polyclonal antibody for gp51 provides
minimal interference with the glycoprotein antigen sites recognised by the
bovine antibodies, ensures optimal presentation of antigen and reduces the
non-specific binding observed with serum from immunised animals, which
often contains antibodies to non-viral antigens. High background values
are observed when BLV antigen is adsorbed directly onto the wells of microtitre plates probably because of the contamination of the BLV preparation
by cellular antigens. Index values (mean value of OD for positive sera
divided by mean value of OD for negative sera at the same dilution)

generally cited in the literature in this case were less than 2.0 (Graves et al., 1982). The use of purified gp51 as antigen in ELISA test would most probably overcome this disadvantage of high non-specific binding but would also significantly increase the cost of the test. Monoclonal antibodies adsorbed to the well specifically select for the antigen contained in a non-purified preparation. Since monoclonal antibody can be produced in unlimited amounts from ascitic fluids, our test thus also provides a cheap method for the detection of anti-BLV antibodies.

Standardisation and reproducibility of ELISA involving monoclonal antibody is very easy since monoclonal antibodies are homogeneous and mono-specific reagents.

For the large scale detection of BLV infection with an ELISA system, it is necessary to automate the ELISA procedure (multiple washings, precision of the dilution, multiple incubation with different reagents) in order to obtain a diagnostic test which would be as practical as the immunodiffusion test for the detection of BLV specific antibodies in sera.

PRESENT AND FUTURE APPLICATIONS

Bovine material is known to be the most complicated material to be used in ELISA techniques because high non-specific binding is frequently observed.

A proper choice of the conditions used in our non-classical ELISA technique for BLV was necessary to render this test sensitive, specific and reproducible. The lack of need for antigen purification also makes this test a cheap test. These important technical considerations are probably also suitable for the large scale detection of other bovine viral antibodies or antigens eg rotaviruses and coronaviruses.

At the present time, the sensitivity of all ELISA tests greatly depends on the avidity of the antibodies used in the conjugate. To reduce the non-specific signal in the bovine system, it is absolutely necessary to use antibodies and more precisely Fab fragments isolated by immunoadsorption.

In the future, the use of conjugates with highly avid monoclonal antibodies directed against several epitopes on the bovine immunoglobulins might obviate the need for polyclonal antibodies isolated by immunoadsorption. Monoclonal antibodies can be utilised in a wide variety of immunoassays eg ELISA, immunofluorescence etc to overcome the disadvantages inherent to the generation of antibodies in animals (presence of non-specific antibodies).

ELISA and monoclonal antibodies technology thus appear as two complementary new developments in veterinary research. This is especially true in BLV research, where they provide a basis for serological surveillance of the cattle population and also for the production of an experimental vaccine. Monoclonal antibodies allow an independent study of each epitope displayed by an antigenic molecule and thus facilitate the study of antigenic variation among different virus isolates as well as the study of an eventual gp51 subunit or a synthetic peptide to be used as a vaccine against BLV infection. BLV-neutralising monoclonal antibodies can be used as probes for the detection of these important epitopes in the development of a BLV vaccine.

APPENDIX

ELISA TEST FOR DETECTION OF BOVINE ANTIBODIES TO BLV

Some modifications were brought to the procedure previously described (Portetelle et al., 1983a).

Monoclonal antibody (100 ng per well) in 50 μl of PBS (pH 7.4; sodium phosphate 0.01 M, NaCl 0.15 M) was incubated for 16 h at 4°C in the wells of a 96-well microtitre plate (GIBCO 2-69620). Unbound antibody was discarded and the wells were washed twice with 200 μl of PBS containing 0.2% Tween 80 (washing buffer). Saturation buffer (50 μl of buffer pH 7.4, sodium phosphate 0.2 M, NaCl 0.15 M containing 2% bovine serum albumin and 0.06% azide) was added into each well; after 15 minutes, 50 μl of culture supernatant from BLV infected cell line was added and mixed. After at least 24 h incubation at 4°C, the antigen solution was discarded and the wells were washed twice with 200 μl of washing buffer. The sera to be tested were diluted (first dilution 1:20, dilution factor 1:3) in 200 μl of reaction buffer (PBS containing 2% bovine serum albumin, 2% Tween 80, 10% glycerol and 0.02% azide) and incubated overnight at 4°C.

The wells were then washed three times with 200 μl of washing buffer and 50 μl of the same buffer containing the POD-Fab or GAL-Fab anti-bovine immunoglobulin conjugate at a concentration of 35 ng Fab per well. The plate was incubated at room temperature for another 4 h and then washed four times with washing buffer. Bound peroxidase was revealed by adding 100 μl of freshly prepared substrate (0.04% chromogenic substrate and

0.02% peroxide) in 0.1 M Na H$_2$ PO$_4$. H$_2$O, pH5. Bound β-galactosidase was revealed by adding 100 µl of freshly prepared substrate (0.08% ONPG) in 0.1 M Na H$_2$ PO$_4$. H$_2$O, pH7, containing 1 mM MgSO$_4$ and 0.2 mM Mn SO$_4$. The mixture was allowed to react for 20 mins at room temperature in the dark (POD) or for 45 mins (GAL). The reaction was stopped by the addition of 100 µl 6N HCl (POD) or 100 µl 1M Na$_2$ CO$_3$ (GAL). The optical density was scored by a Microelisa Automatic Reader.

REFERENCES

Altaner, C., Zajac, V. and Ban, J. 1982. Zbl. Vet. Med. B., 29, 583-590.
Avrameas, S. 1983. Current Topics Micr. Immun., 104, 93-99.
Bruck, C., Portetelle, D., Glineur, C. and Bollen, A. 1982a. J. Immunol. Methods, 53, 313-319.
Bruck, C., Mathot, S., Portetelle, D., Berte, C., Franssen, J.D., Herion,P. and Burny, A. 1982b. Virology, 122, 342-352.
Bruck, C., Portetelle, D., Burny, A. and Zavada, J. 1982c. Virology, 122, 353-362.
Bruck, C., Portetelle, D., Burny, A. and Zavada, J. 1983. In "Current Topics in Veterinary Medicine and Animal Science" (Ed. O.C. Straub). (Martinus Nijhoff, The Hague), in press.
Burny, A., Bruck, C., Chantrenne, H., Cleuter, G., Dekegel, D., Ghysdaep J., Kettmann, R., Leclercq, M., Leunen, J., Mammerickx, M. and Portetelle, D. 1980. In "Viral Oncology" (Ed. G. Klein). (Raven Press, New York). pp. 231-289.
De Savigny, D. and Voller, A. 1980. In "Immunoenzymatic Assay Techniques" (Ed. R. Malvano) (Martinus Nijhoff, The Hague). pp. 116-148.
Graves, D.C., McQuade, M. and Weibel, K. 1982. Am. J. Vet. Res., 43, 960-966.
Hoff-Jorgensen, R. 1980. In "CEC Scientific Workshop on Bovine Leukosis" (Ed. L.M. Markson). (ECSC-EEC-EAEC, Brussels-Luxembourg). pp. 55-66.
Langone,J.J.and Van Vunakis, H. 1983. Immunochemical techniques. Part E. Monoclonal antibodies and general immunoassay methods. Meth. Enzymol., 92, 647 p.
Mammerickx, M., Cormann, A., Burny, A., Dekegel, D. and Portetelle, D. 1978. Ann. Rech. Vet., 9, 885-894.
Mammerickx, M., Portetelle, D., Burny, A. and Leunen, J. 1980. Zbl. Vet. Med. B., 27, 291-303.
Mammerickx, M., Portetelle, D., Bruck, C. and Burny, A. 1983. Zbl. Vet. Med. B., 30, in press.
Manz, D., Wiegand, D., Behrens, F. and Ziegelmaier, R. 1981. Zbl. Vet. Med. B., 28, 280-291.
Maris, P., Nougayrede, P.H. and Perrin, G. 1983. Comp. Immun. Microbiol. Infect. Dis., 6, 45-50.
O'Sullivan, M.J. and Marks, V. 1981. In "Methods in Enzymology". Vol. 73. (Eds. J.J. Langone and H. Van Vunakis). (Academic Press, New York). pp. 747-766.
Portetelle, D., Bruck, C., Mammerickx, M. and Burny, A. 1980. Virology, 105, 223-233.
Portetelle, D., Bruck, C., Mammerickx, M. and Burny, A. 1983a. J. Virol. Methods, 6, 19-29.

Portetelle, D., Bruck, C., Mammerickx, M. and Burny, A. 1983b. In "Current topics in Veterinary Medicine and Animal Science" (Ed. O.C. Straub). (Martinus Nijhoff, The Hague), in press.

Ressang, A.A., Gielkens, A.L.J., Quak, J. and Mastenbroek, N. 1980. In "CEC Scientific Workshop on Bovine Leukosis" (Ed. L.M. Markson). (ECSC-EEC-EAEC, Brussels-Luxembourg). pp. 67-80.

Van Der Maaten, M.J. and Miller, J. 1976. Bibl. Haematol., 43, 360-362.

Yolken, R.H. 1983. Current Topics Micr. Immun., 104, 177-194.

RADIOIMMUNOASSAY

Daniel Levy

INSERM U 152 Hopital Cochin - 27 rue du fg Saint Jacques
75014 Paris, France

ABSTRACT

Radioimmunoassay is an analytical method based upon the labelling of a purified antigen. It offers a combination of convenience, specificity and sensitivity, but requires the use of an inconvenient separation step. Conversely, labelled (radioactive or not) antibody techniques suffer from higher non-specific binding, but appear more convenient and may be improved in sensitivity.

INTRODUCTION

The measurement of picograms (10^{-12} g) of an antigen is relatively simple, precise and rapid if the antigen is radioactively labelled. The scope and precision obtained by the use of labelled antigens for the study of antigen-antibody reactions is considerable and their use has been elaborated from the initial discovery by Yalow and Berson (1960) into a well-established system, the radioimmunoassay (RIA). This method offers a unique combination of specificity, sensitivity, precision and practicality for the microdetermination of specific proteins in unfractionated mixtures.

When a labelled antigen is used it is only this label which is measured. At the concentration used the Ag : Ab complex remains in solution, though in most cases the systems would show precipitation at higher concentrations. The reaction of the labelled Ag with antibody can be followed and the system analysed if a method is available for the separation of the antibody-bound labelled antigen from the free labelled antigen. This separation may be achieved by exploiting differences in molecular size, charge, adsorption or solubility properties of the two moieties or by precipitation of the bound antigen using a second antibody raised to the globulin of the first antibody.

GENERAL PRINCIPLES

All methods of measurement of substances in biological fluids entail reaction between the substance to be measured and some form of "analytical reagent". The term "immunoassay" is commonly applied to analytical methods in which the analytical reagent is a specific antibody capable of binding to the substance to be measured (antigen). The basic principles underlying all such analytical methods, including immunoassay techniques, are independent of the nature of the specific reagent used and fall into two broad categories: "antigen-observed" and "antibody-observed" techniques. These descriptions refer to the fact that the analytical reaction can be examined by observation, in the first case, of the fate of the antigen following reaction and, in the second of the antibody.

The distinction drawn between these two analytical approaches is not a trivial one: the basic performance characteristics of assays falling into each category, their sensitivity, their specificity, and the speed with which they can be performed are essentially dissimilar.

"Radioimmunoassay" constitutes the classic example of an "antigen-observed" analytical procedure. This general method fundamentally relies on a binding reaction between the antigen and a specific antibody. Radiolabelled antigen is added to the reaction to act as an "indicator" to the final distribution of the unlabelled antigen between the two compartments (the labelled antigen is neither required to be chemically identical to, nor to be introduced into the reaction system together with, the unlabelled antigen and is not therefore necessarily a true tracer of the latter in the antigen reaction) (Fig.1).

"Immunoradiometric assay" is the term which is usually applied to those immunoassays which, whilst also utilising radio-labelling techniques, fall into the category "antibody-observed" analytical methods. Thus, in contrast to RIA, these techniques rely on observation of the distribution of the antibody and it is the antibody reagent which is therefore radiolabelled in this type of method. As is analogously the case in the labelled antigen methods, the labelled antibody serves as an indicator of the final distribution of the antibody following the reaction, but it is likewise not essential that the labelled antibody molecule should be chemically identical to any unlabelled antibody molecules that may also be present in the preparation (Fig.1).

Although this system and its variants employ the same reagents and techniques as RIA, they are fundamentally different. RIA is a form of isotope dilution analysis, the specific binding reagent is used at a limited concentration and need not be monospecific since only those antibodies which bind the tracer are involved. In the IRMA system the antibody is used essentially to prepare a labelled derivative whose molar concentration is

Radioimmunoassay (RIA)

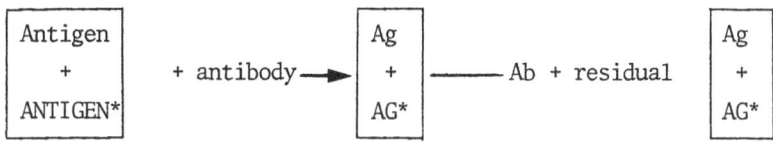

Observation of the final distribution of labelled AG* between complex and residuum.

Immunoradiometric assay (IRMA)

Observation of the final distribution of labelled AB* between complex and residuum.

Fig. 1   RIA and IRMA.

proportional to, and ideally is identical with, the molar concentration of antigen in the unknown. The labelled antibody can therefore be added in excess to force the reaction, although this will tend to increase the relative potency of cross-reacting substances. The labelled antibody must be monospecific and consequently its preparation includes an immunosorbent step. In theory, the molar detection limit of this system would be the same as the molar detection limit of ^{125}I ie about 10 attamole (1×10^{-19} g). In practice non-specific reactions build serious inroads into this and IRMA detection limits are of about the same order as RIA. It seems likely that special considerations may lead to a preference for IRMA, eg when the antigen is unstable and/or poses special problems for iodination.

In the "sandwich" or two-sites IRMA the analytical reaction between antigen and labelled antibody is essentially combined with an immuno-extraction step, in which the antigen is extracted from the test sample by an immuno-adsorbent, ie by an "extraction" antibody coupled to a solid support (Fig. 2).

THE RADIOIMMUNOASSAY (RIA)

174

A. Labelling proteins and polypeptides

The ability of RIA to measure picogram quantities can be exploited only if the antigen can be labelled to high specific activity. While labelling of proteins with tritium or ^{14}C- acetyl groups has occasionally been used, there has been widespread reliance on the use of radioiodine. As generally used, one atom of ^{125}I offers approximately two counts for every one count given by an atom of ^{131}I. The specific activity of a ^{125}I- protein having one atom iodine per molecule is approximately 100 μCi/μg at a mol wt. of 20 000 and 1 000 μCi/μg at 2 000 mol wt.

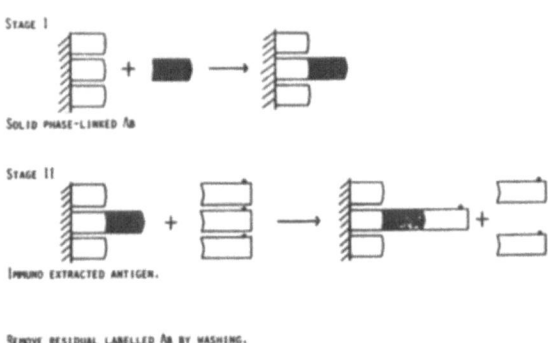

Fig.2   The "sandwich" immunoradiometric assay. In the first stage analyte is sequestered on to solid-phased antibody. The second stage involves reaction between "immuno-extracted" antigen and labelled antibody.

The chemistry of radio-iodination is essentially the chemistry of substitution of iodine into tyrosine groups. Iodine monochloride (ICl) facilitates a maximum possible iodine utilization of 100 per cent.

The direct iodination of proteins can be done by different ways.

1.Chloramine - T procedure: almost universally used
   - very low concentrations of reagent
   - very small quantities of protein (1-5 μg)
   - separation of the iodinated protein from unreacted iodide and other low mol. wt. reactants rapidly achieved by means of gel filtration
   - optimum pH = 7.4
   - yield of iodination
     100% at concentration of protein >1 mg/ml
     80-90% at concentration of protein 300 μg/ml

60-70% at concentration of protein 50 µg/ml

2. We have been using since several years an oxidative step utilizing
the IODOGEN (Pierce) procedure:
- advantages: . all reactants ready
                     . no need of additional substances to stop the
                       oxidizing process
                     . same yields of iodination as chloramine T.

- disadvantage: . immunologic activity of glycoproteins slight-
                       ly altered.

3. Conjugation labelling: Bolton and Hunter (1972)
Iodination by chloramine - T method of a small molecule, that binds
to amino-acids (NH_2 of lysine or N-terminal) of the proteins via a
peptide bond.
- advantages: . protein not exposed to oxidizing or reducing
                       agents
                     . means of introducing iodine into proteins
                       lacking tyrosine
                     . antigenic determinants involving tyrosine are
                       not affected.

- disadvantages: . modification of some amino groups of the
                       antigen
                     . manipulations slightly more complex.

B. Selection of diluent solution

In general RIA work involves manipulations of antigen (Ag) and labelled antigen (* Ag) at low concentrations and serious losses by adsorption
to glass or plastic vessels and consequent non-specific effects are encountered unless these losses are eliminated. Assay diluent consists usually of buffer (eg 0.05 Mol/l pH 7.5) to which is added a suitable carrier
protein. For this purpose 2 per cent animal protein or serum is generally
suitable but this should be checked for each new antigen. The following
factors should be considered:
1. The protein content should be adequate to completely prevent adsorption of * Ag at the lowest concentration being considered.
2. If animal serum is used it should be free of Ag and of any possible

176

cross-reacting substances.

3. A bacteriostatic agent, eg sodium azide 0.1 g/litre may be incorporated.

4. The stability of * Ag in the diluent: both Ag and more particularly * Ag may show limited stability at the low concentrations used and this can be important especially when incubation times are extended in order to achieve maximum sensitivity.

C. Separation of antibody-bound from free labelled antigen

In the systems under consideration only labelled antigen is determined and the reaction with antibody may be investigated if the labelled antigen bound to antibody can be separated from the unreacted "free" antigen. This separation may be achieved either physicochemically or by means of a second immunological step.

1.The double-antibody method. The antibody complexed to the labelled antigen is precipitated by anti-ɣ- globulin raised in a second species. In the radioimmunoassay the primary antigen-antibody complex is too dilute to be precipitated; however, if carrier non-immune serum belonging to the same species as the first antibody is first added and this is followed by an antiserum raised in a second species to the ɣ - globulin of the first antibody a sizeable lattice can be built up and the whole, including the labelled antigen bound to the first antibody, can be precipitated. The method gives excellent separations (1-3 per cent apparent bound in the absence of antibody and ⟩95 per cent bound in excess antibody), can handle any convenient volume of incubate if carefully optimized, is unaffected by variations in (plasma) protein concentration and is gentle, simple, and well suited to handling very large numbers of tubes. A single experiment is sufficient to optimize a double-antibody system with a given second antiserum and once this has been completed for one antigen identical conditions may well be found to be suitable for a large number of other antigens, provided the same species is used to raise the first antibody in each case.

Examples of experiments designed to find the optimum conditions for a double-antibody system (Hunter, 1978) are shown in Fig 3.

The double-antibody method would appear to suffer from only two disadvantages:

1. Cost.

2. The second antibody generally cannot be used in high dilution and
a large pool of serum is required to sustain the high output of an
active radioimmunoassay laboratory.

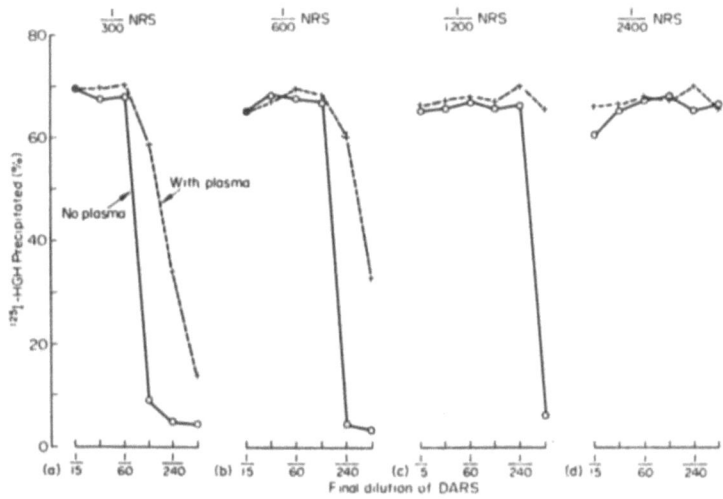

Fig. 3   Optimal conditions for a double-antibody system, with a
donkey anti-rabbit- γ-globulin serum (DARS) for human growth hormone.
The same mixture of ^{125}I-HGH and rabbit anti-HGH antiserum (first
antibody) was used. Carrier normal rabbit serum (NRS) at different
dilutions was tested. Precipitation still complete with NRS used at
1:2 400 and unaffected by antigen-free plasma. DARS chosen at 1:120.

2.SaC.I precipitation. We developed and have used since 1976 a second
step precipitation utilizing the property of Protein-A, present on the membrane of Staphylococcus aureus Cowan I, to bind to the Fc fragment of mammalian immunoglobulins G (Levy et al., 1977). As illustrated in Fig.4, the
final precipitation of the immune complexes is identical to that obtained
with a second antibody. In addition, the SaC.I precipitation:
   - is more rapid to perform
   - allows a complete precipitation at any dilution of the first serum
   - is free of non-specific binding
   - is of very low cost if home-made
   - but it reacts only with mammalian IgG antibodies.

D.   The use of labelled antigen
   1. Detection of antibodies. The equilibration time is a function of the

178

concentration of Ag and Ab and of the energy of the reaction. The energy
of the reaction is a function of the "avidity" of the antiserum.

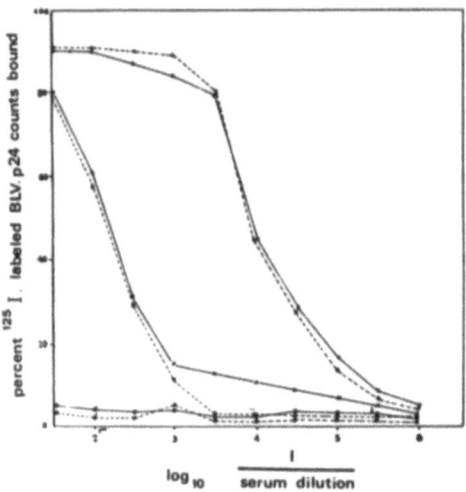

Fig. 4   RIA titration curves. Labelled BLV p24 was incubated with
varying dilutions of sera. Three different sera were used: 1) serum
No 531 from a lymphocytotic cow precipitated by undiluted rabbit anti-
bovine immunoglobulin serum (•-----•) or by the SaCI preparation
(•————•); 2) serum of normal cow from a leukemia-free and non-BLV
exposed herd precipitated by undiluted rabbit anti-bovine immunoglobulin serum (■-----■) or by the SaCI preparation (■————■); and
3) goat serum anti-BLV; the final precipitation being done either by
undiluted rabbit anti-goat immunoglobulin serum (x -----x) or by the
SaCI preparation (x ———— x).

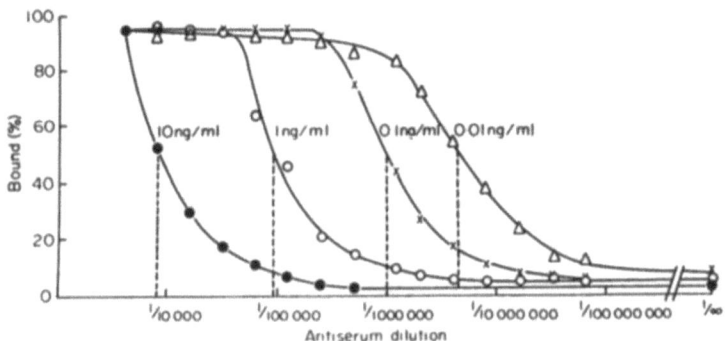

Fig. 5   Antiserum titration curve: one anti-insulin serum titrated
against 4 different concentrations of ^{125}I-insulin.

Fig.5 shows curves for a single antiserum titrated against four different concentrations of Ag. The three curves to the left representing 10 ng/ml, 1 ng/ml and 0.1 ng/ml ^{125}I-Ag are parallel, and perpendicular through 50% binding at antiserum dilutions of approximately 10^{-4}, 10^{-5} and 10^{-6}, ie show ten-fold differences in antiserum dilution. The fourth curve fails to show the full displacement. This lack of proportionality is caused by failure of Ag and Ab to react in this attenuated dilution. The antiserum used was of very high avidity, able to distinguish between 0.1 and 0.01 ng/ml.

Another property of the antiserum is illustrated in the same figure: the titre, which represents the quantity of Ab in the antiserum. Convenient comparisons between antisera may be made by using an arbitrary definition of titre, eg dilution of antibody required to bind 50% or a lower percentage of the labelled Ag. Strictly, it is necessary to show that, at the concentration of Ag used to determine the titre, the antiserum is still in the area of proportionality and that the labelled Ag has the same affinity as cold Ag for the particular antiserum under test.

2.Antigen addition curves: the RIA. If a mixture of * Ag and sufficient antibody to bind about 50% of this label is incubated with serial dilutions of cold Ag, then hot and cold Ag will compete for the limited number of binding sites on the available antibody. There will be a sequential fall in per cent bound through the series. If unlabelled Ag is plotted on a log-scale, the regression becomes linear over a certain range. This forms the basis of the RIA.

Standard curve: A standard curve has certain characteristics which affect the precision, sensitivity and working range of the assay. In Fig.6, the following factors emerge: the percentage of labelled Bovine Leukemia Virus p24 (used at 0.5 ng in each sample) bound to antibody in the absence of added unlabelled Ag is 70%. Addition of an equal amount of unlabelled Ag (0.5 ng p24 in 1 ng total virus) equal to the concentration of the labelled Ag results in a fall of 10 in the per cent bound (ie an increase of 10% in the displacement of bound labelled Ag). This variation is the result of doubling the concentration of the total antigen (labelled + cold p24) and is about the same as the slope (variation in per cent bound per doubling dose of standard) of the standard curve. In conclusion:

- the dilution of Ab is optimal for the concentration of labelled Ag

used,
- labelled Ag shows no loss of affinity for the Ab.

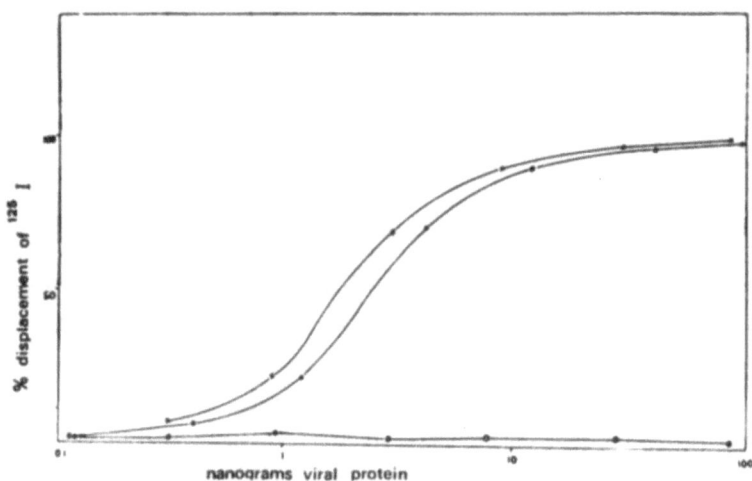

Fig.6   Competitive RIA for BLV p24. Detergent-disrupted viruses
were used as competing antigens and were mixed with a concentration
of serum No 531 known to precipitate approximately 50% of the labelled antigen 1:4,000. x ——— x BLV from FLS; •———• BLV from
FLK; o ———o Mol.MuLV.

The percentage of label bound can be increased by using a higher concentration of antiserum. However, this takes the system above the central
linear part of the range and the fall in per cent bound for the first standard is reduced, ie the sensitivity of the assay is impaired. A reduction
in the concentration of antiserum is less serious and merely results in a
lower percentage bound for the "0" standard and a shortening of the working
range of the assay. The mean slope in the example given is steep enough to
give a high order of precision but not so steep that the effective working
range is restricted.

DISCUSSION

A.   RIA sensitivity

Sensitivity is the lower limit of detection or, its essential equivalent, the precision of measurement of zero dose. The following parameters
govern the ultimate sensitivity attainable with a conventional RIA:
    1. equilibrium constant of the Ab/Ag reaction

2. experimental error in the measurement of the distribution of labelled Ag between Ab-bound and free moieties
3. specific activity of the labelled Ag
4. extent of misclassification of bound and free moieties (non-
   specific binding of labelled Ag to Ab).

In practice, the specific activities of the radioactively labelled Ag
employed in the majority of RIA procedures are such as not to constitute a
major constraint on assay sensitivity. Thus the principal limitations are
imposed by the experimental errors arising in the determination of the
assay response variable and the equilibrium constant of the antibody/anti-
gen reaction. The misclassification of bound and free moieties also affects
assay sensitivity; however, the influence of this factor on the assay detection limit per se is also, in practice, relatively minor. Thus, although
each of the four factors listed above influences the sensitivity of an RIA
procedure, the equilibrium constant and the "experimental" errors in the
measurement of the response variable are, in practice, dominant (Table 1).

Note that a reverse situation exists for IRMA where specific activity
and non-specific binding are more important (Table 1).

TABLE 1   Factors affecting the sensitivity of RIA and IRMA

	RIA	IRMA
Specific Activity	+	++++
Non-specific binding	+	++++
Equilibrium constant	++++	+
Experimental errors	++++	+
Optimal amount Ab	→ 0	→ ∞

B. RIA specificity

Assay non-specificity in immunoassay procedures arises in consequence
of two main causes:

   a) the existence in test samples of cross-reactants capable of react-
      ing with the antibody reagent.
   b) the existence of other substances (salts, urea, etc.) which in-
      fluence the avidity of the antigen/antibody reaction.

A cross-reactant in a labelled antigen assay system "competes" with the
Ag for the limited number of antibody binding sites and thus effectively

simulates the Ag in affecting the distribution of labelled Ag between free and antibody-bound moieties. However, under assay conditions which yield maximal assay sensitivity (ie (Ab)→0), the relative potency of the cross-reactant vis-a-vis the Ag tends towards, and approximates to, a value given by the ratio of the avidities (ie equilibrium constants) of the two substances with respect to the antibody binding sites. This implies that a cross-reactant which, for example, reacts ten times less avidly than the Ag with specific antibody binding sites will display a relative potency in the assay system of approximately 1/10th and a 10-fold larger amount of cross-reactant than of Ag will be required to exert an equal effect in the assay system.

In RIA, both Ag and Ab are generally present at very low concentrations. So, the distribution of antigen between free and bound fractions is very dependent on the value of K, and any changes in K arising from the presence in incubation mixtures of components which alter the thermodynamic constants of the binding reaction will lead to marked non-specific effects on antigen measurements.

CONCLUSION

An increasing interest has been displayed in the development of analytical methods which, whilst retaining the characteristics of convenience, specificity and sensitivity possessed by radioimmunoassay might offer particular improvements with regard to one or other of these attributes. For example, much effort has been expended in the search for non-isotopic labels which might be substituted for radioisotopes either on grounds associated with the use of radioactivity, or for reasons relating to cost and general inconvenience of instrumentation and reagents; the principal disadvantages associated with radiolabelled reagents have centred on their inevitably limited shelf life, and on the fact that, in practice, their use in analytical procedures such as RIA requires an inconvenient "separation step". Much skill and ingenuity has therefore been expended in attempting to develop non-isotopic techniques which would eliminate the disadvantages associated with radioassay methods.

In practice, the gains in convenience deriving from the use of non-isotopic methods - particularly those which endeavour to avoid the physical separation stage characteristic of the radioisotopic methods - have tended to be accompanied by significant loss in sensitivity. This has implied that the exploitation of non-isotopic labels has been largely confined to substances which are present in biological fluids at relatively high concentration, and they have not offered a serious challenge to conventional RIA for the measurement of those substances for which the RIA and related methods were primarily introduced.

Finally, since the labelled Ag techniques are not currently constrained in sensitivity by the specific activity of radioisotopes such as I^{125}, no increase in assay sensitivity can be anticipated in such Ag procedures by the use of alternative labelling techniques. Indeed, in general, the use of other forms of label usually, though not inevitably, generates additional forms of error in the measurement of the response variable which results in significant losses in assay sensitivity.

Conversely, since the assay sensitivities of labelled antibody techniques can, in certain circumstances, be limited by the specific activity of currently available labels, it is in this type of analytical approach that alternative forms of label, which display much higher specific activities than radioisotopic markers, can be expected ultimately to lead to significant improvements in sensitivity over that attainable by present radioimmunoassay methods.

TECHNICAL APPENDIX

I. Iodination of proteins.

1. Optional: take 5 drops conc. potassium iodine solution one hour prior to iodination to block thyroid uptake.

2. Prepare column (see below*).

3. Purified protein to be iodinated is stored frozen in 10 λ aliquots (10 micrograms).

4. Add 25 λ of (0.4M Tris pH 7.4, 4mM EDTA) buffer to purified protein.

5. a) Prepare chloramine T (25 mg/10 ml 0.01M Tris, 0.01M NaCl). Solution must be fresh.

    b) Prepare sodium meta bisulfite (25 mg/10 ml 0.01M NaCl). Solution must be fresh.

    c) In iodination hood add 10 λ (1 mCi) ^{125}I to protein. Immediately add 10 λ chloramine T and time reaction with stopwatch for one minute. Shake reaction mixture for just 30 seconds of reaction time. Chloramine T is used to oxidize the protein molecule so that the iodine can attach to it.

d) At end of 1 min. immediately add 25 λ of sodium meta bisulfite ($Na_2S_2O_5$) to stop reaction.

6. Iodogen procedure.

   a) Preparation of Iodogen.

      - Dissolve in a glass tube 10 mg Iodogen in 1 ml Chloroform. Keep on ice.

      - Aliquote in glass tubes by 20 µl.

      - Briefly lyophilyse, or evaporate under fume hood.

      - Store at -20°.

   b) For labelling, thaw one iodogen tube at room temperature.

   c) Sequentially add in iodination hood:

      - protein to be iodinated (with 25 µl 0.4M Tris-HCl pH 7.4, 0.01M NaCl).

      - 1 mCi ^{125}I.

   d) Time reaction for one minute, and gently mix with Pasteur pipette.

7. Use Pasteur Pipette to remove reaction mixture and add gently to column. Rinse reaction vial with buffer[+] and add to column. After this has gone into gel bed move column to next tube and fill to top with buffer[+]. Collect 0.5 ml fractions.

8. Count each fraction in well counter. Pool peak, up to 3 fractions in siliconized tube. Add equal volume of buffer I (from Radio-immune-precipitation assay) and store at 4^oC.

Preparation of Column 1) Ready to use PD.10 (Pharmacia). 2) Bio Rad p10 suspended in buffer[+]; allowed to swell. Use 10 ml plastic pipette with top cut off as column. Place 2" rubber tubing on bottom and glass beads inside pipette. Pour gel in the column, allow to pack.

Add 1.5 ml of 2% ovalbumin and wash several times with buffer[+].

+ Buffer column and elution: 0.01M Tris pH 7.8, 0.01M NaCl.

11. Radioimmunoassay procedure.

Solutions:

A. Buffer I

BSA	2 %
NaN3	0.1 %
EDTA	0.003 M
Tris pH 7.8	0.01 M
Triton X-100	0.7 %
NaCl	0.01 M

Make up to 1 litre and adjust pH to 7.8.

B. Buffer II

Tris pH 7.8   0.01 M
NaCl   0.01 M
Triton X-100 0.1 %

Make up to 1 litre.

Rinse buffer: 0.01 M Tris pH 7.8, 0.1% Triton
0.1 M NaCl, 0.001 M EDTA

Radioimmunoprecipitation Assay for Detecting Antibodies in Sera to BLV.

1. Make sera dilutions in 50 µl buffer I. (1/30 - 1/100 - 1/300 - 1/1000 - ... - $1/10^6$: 23 µl of 1/30 in 50 µl buffer I. Mix. Transfer 23 µl of mixture to second tube).

2. Add 100 µl Buffer II to each tube.

3. Prepare ^{125}I-Ag in buffer I to have approximately 10,000 CPM/50 µl. Add 50 µl to each tube.

4. Incubate at 37°C for 3 hours and 4° overnight.

5. Add 50 µl of antibody 2 (goat or rabbit anti-IgG) to each tube, or 75 µl of 10% SAC. I.

6. Incubate at 37°C for 1 hr and at 4°C for 3 hrs (2^d antibody), or at 4°C for 15 mins (SAC. I).

7. Add 0.4 ml rinse buffer to all tubes.

8. Centrifuge at 2,500 rpm for 15 mins.

9. Aspirate the supernatant, measure the radioactivity in the pellet.

REFERENCES

Bolton, A.E. and Hunter, W.M. 1972. A new method for labelling protein hormones with radioiodine for use in the radioimmunoassay. J. Endocrinol., 55, xxx-xxxi.
Hunter, W.M. 1978. In "Handbook of Experimental Immunology". 3rd Edition. (Blackwell Scientific Publications).
Levy, D., Deshayes, L., Parodi, A.L., Levy, J.P., Stephenson, J.R., Devare, S.G. and Gilden, R.V. 1977. Bovine leukemia virus specific antibodies among French cattle. II. Radioimmunoassay with the major structural protein (BLV p24). Int. J. Cancer, 20, 543-550.
Yalow, R.S. and Berson, S.A. 1960. Immunoassay of endogenous plasma insulin in man. J. Clin. Invest, 39, 1157-1163.

IMMUNOELECTROPHORETIC TECHNIQUES

K. Dalsgaard

State Veterinary Institute for Virus Research,
Lindholm, DK-4771 Kalvehave, Denmark

ABSTRACT

"Practical and theoretical aspects of immunoelectrophoretic techniques applied to veterinary virus diagnosis are discussed. Included are counter current electrophoresis, rocket electrophoresis, and crossed immunoelectrophoresis. Aspects of the latter technique comprises the production of specific antisera to individual viral antigens".

INTRODUCTION

Immunoelectrophoretic techniques (IT's) are all based on classical precipitation reactions between antigen (ag) and antibody (ab). They are so to say immunodiffusions "speeded up" by electrical current. IT's are practically all carried out in agarose gels. Other supporting media, cellulose strips etc. have been used, but the availability now of agaroses with well defined electroendosmosis has practically excluded other media. The classical immunoelectrophoresis has been reviewed so extensively ever since its introduction by Grabar and Williams in 1953, that it has been omitted in this report. Included are more recent methods with a diagnostic potential: counter current electrophoresis (CC) (also called immunoelectroosmophoresis IEOP), rocket electrophoresis (RE), and crossed immunoelectrophoresis (CIE). The first two techniques are suitable for mass screening, and the latter can be used for the production of "mono"-specific antisera in experimental animals. Many sophisticated variants of immunoelectrophoresis (line electrophoresis, crossed line electrophoresis, fused rockets, tandem crossed electrophoresis etc.) have been published. These techniques are mainly used in research for the comparison of ag or ab. For details the reader is kindly asked to consult the book by Axelsen et al. (1973). This excellent manual, written by a research team at the Protein Laboratory, The University of Copenhagen, covers almost all aspects of immunoelectrophoresis, including equipment, instructive pictures, and full technical details.

In the following I shall restrict myself to consider the practical and theoretical points I have found of importance for the use of immunoelectrophoresis in veterinary virus diagnosis.

CASTING A GEL

Most commonly used agaroses make a suitable gel when used in 1% concentration in buffer. We have found it convenient to store aliquots of 15 ml of gel in test tubes covered with Parafilm. When sodium azide is added to the buffer such gels can be stored for months in the coldroom. When used they are first melted in a boiling water bath and then transferred to a thermostat bath at 56°C. It is important that the tubes are kept here for some minutes to equilibrate. Not only does this temperature permit the addition of antisera, it will also ensure uniform casting conditions from plate to plate. We always use 10 x 10 cm plates. With 15 ml of gel this gives a layer thickness of 1.5 mm. We never use frames and spacers for casting, but simply pour the gel on the horizontal plates. Holes are punched in the gel after congelation. For routine work it is definitely important to possess a good template and a few special gel punchers as described by Axelsen et al. (1973). These small ingenious tools, which cut and suck up the gel bung in one action make an otherwise tedious task extremely easy.

RUNNING A GEL

Any simple electrophoresis apparatus may be used with good results, provided it has a good cooling plate to remove the heat inevitably generated. Usually water cooling is used, and running tap water may be applied. However, better results can be obtained by using a circulating cooling thermostat. Running tap water is normally too cold for the purpose (about 10°C). When the plates become that cold, condensation of water may take place on the gel surface, leading to alteration of the gel buffer and possibly distortion of the ag/ab precipitates. A cooling temperature of 18°C will eliminate this problem.

No two immunoelectrophoresis buffers described in the literature are the same; many substances have been added to facilitate precipitation, clarify the gel etc. There are 3 major requirements to be fulfilled: 1. The pH should normally be 8.6 because most immunoglobulin (IgG) molecules are electrically neutral at this pH. 2. The buffering capacity should be high enough to maintain the pH in the gel throughout the electrophoresis. 3. On the other hand the ionic strength should be as low as possible to avoid excessive heat generation. These requirements are usually met with the following buffer:

Barbital sodium	20.6 g
Barbital	4.0 g
Sodium azide	1.0 g
Distilled water	to make 5 litres.

A stock solution, 5 times concentrated may conveniently be stored. Sodium azide is added to prevent microbial growth. This standard buffer may be used in almost all immunoelectrophoretic systems. It is used to make the gel, and in the electrode vessels. After a typical run the pH in the anodic vessel has risen with about 0.5 pH. For this reason the buffer is discarded after each run.

For electrical contact between the buffer and the gel a variety of materials have been applied. Obviously agarose gel slabs of the same composition as on the plates are excellent but not practical. We always use 3 layers of Whatman no. 1 filter paper cut to 10 x 10 cm. When cut you can ask the manufacturer to indicate the fibre direction. The fibre direction is then placed parallel to the direction of the electrical current. The wick is thoroughly wetted with buffer and the edge gently tapped on the edge of the agarose plate. One should use gloves at this stage - naked fingertips leave more protein on the wick than you like to believe.

When applying the samples to the gels it is advisable to put on a small electrical current (Caution ! small enough to avoid hazards). This minimizes radial diffusion. Then the voltage is increased using a rectifier in the constant voltage mode. The voltage drop per cm gel is the only true value which can be used for standardization of conditions. It should be checked using a voltmeter equipped with two platinum needle electrodes placed exactly 4 cm apart. By gently dipping the electrodes in the gel the meter will show the voltage/cm x 4.

For a quick electrophoresis in the system described the plates are adjusted to 10 V/cm and the electrophoresis run for 2.5 h. Often it is more convenient to run rockets and counter currents overnight, and the voltage is then adjusted to 1.5 V/cm.

STAINING A GEL

Our regular staining procedure takes less than 3 hours and comprises the following:

A piece of dry Whatman 3 M filter paper is placed on top of the gel avoiding air bubbles. A gentle pressure (filter pads and a glass plate) is put on. After 15 mins the gel will be squeezed flat like a sponge. The paper is removed and the plates are placed in a rack. The plates are now left to soak for 2 x 10 mins in 0.85% NaCl, and 1 x 10 mins in distilled water. The paper squeezing step is repeated, and the plates are now dried in a hot air stream for 30 mins. We use one of the common 1-2 kW household heating blowers available everywhere. The agarose layer will now be extremely thin and almost invisible. We used to stain our plates in Coomassie brilliant blue containing 40% methanol and 10% acetic acid. But with the increasing awareness of the possible health damaging properties of organic solvents in mind, we have switched to an aqueous based non-biohazardous stain (Crowle and Cline, 1977):

Crocein scarlet	2.5 g
Brilliant blue R	0.15 g
Acetic acid	50 g
Trichloroacetic acid	30 g
Distilled water	to make 1 litre

The plates are left for 30 mins in this staining solution. Destaining only requires a 2 min dip in 0.3% acetic acid followed by a rinse in distilled water. The plates are finally dried in the hot air stream.

ELECTROENDOSMOSIS

To make proper use of the different types of agaroses available, it is necessary to understand the phenomenon of electroendosmosis (EEO). EEO in agarose gels occurs because some of the agaroses contain negatively charged (sulphate) groups. During electrophoresis such groups will tend to move towards the positive electrode. Since the groups are fixed in the gel structure this is not possible. To compensate for this a flow of water towards the negative electrode takes place. So, for practical purposes the only thing we need to know about electroendosmosis is that it causes a cathodic backflow - high when the net number of negatively charged groups in the agarose is high, and low or negligible when the net number is low. In fact the system can be regarded as a small electrical pump, slowly pumping water from the positive to the negative electrode vessel.

It follows from this, that an electrically neutral substance applied to the gel will be moved downstream, towards the cathode. This is the basis of counter current electrophoresis.

COUNTER CURRENT ELECTROPHORESIS (CC)

CC can be used for the screening of serum samples for antibodies against a given virus. In CC-gels two holes are punched approximately 15 mm apart. The serum sample or dilutions of it is placed in the anodic well and the (viral) antigen in the cathodic well. During electrophoresis the ideal situation is that ab moves towards the cathode, and the ag towards the anode eventually forming a precipitate when they meet. When the above-mentioned buffer pH 8.6 is used most of the ab will be electrically neutral. To move the antibody towards the cathode an agarose of relatively high electroendosmosis is needed eg type LSA, Litex, Glostrup, Denmark. Fortunately most antigens are highly negatively charged at pH 8.6, ie their isoelectric point is lower than that of IgG. Therefore the ag will normally move towards the anode. To meet the ab it has to move upstream against the cathodic backflow, ie counter the current.

Having these principles in mind, it is relatively easy to establish a CC system for a given ag/ab system by a series of simple experiments. Choosing an agarose with lower electroendosmosis eg Litex type HSA, HSB, or even HSC will decrease the cathodic backflow and move the precipitation area closer to the ab well. Decreasing the pH of the buffer system will increase the number of ab's with a positive charge, thus making them move faster towards the cathode. A decrease in pH will also slow down the migration of ag towards the anode, but not necessarily at the same rate.

By a combination of these parameters it is usually possible to establish a system that works. Most of the enteroviruses and parvoviruses are good candidates. So are the enveloped RNA and DNA viruses. With enveloped viruses we have found it useful to work with antigens split with non-ionic detergents, but systems without detergent have been published by others. When using detergents it is important to incorporate the detergent eg 1% Triton X-100 throughout the electrophoretic system, ie in the gel, in the wicks, and in the buffer vessels to avoid gradients.

Not all viral ag's have a sufficiently low isoelectric point to be suitable for CC. We have had difficulties using the technique with bovine viral diarrhoea virus, and foot-and-mouth disease virus.

In the oral presentation examples will be given where CC has been used successfully eg porcine parvovirus (Sørensen et al.,1980), swine vesicular disease (Sørensen, 1980), Aujeszky's disease (Dalsgaard, 1982), hog cholera (Terpstra and van Oirschot, 1975), and African swine fever (Pan et al.,1972).

Like in most other serological systems the specificity of the test depends on the purification of the antigen. Where possible, density gradient purified virus is preferable, but in general the plates can be easily read. False positives are rare and may be checked by comparison of the serum sample with a hyperimmune serum using the modified Kohn's test as described by Sørensen (1980). The sensitivity of the test is in general higher than immunodiffusion tests but lower than ELISA and neutralisation tests. As a screening test for serum samples taken on a herd basis the test is sufficiently sensitive. It is used extensively for Aleutian disease (Cho and Ingram, 1972), African swine fever (Pan et al., 1972) and swine vesicular disease (Sørensen, 1980).

ROCKET ELECTROPHORESIS (RE)

RE is used for the screening of samples (faeces, body fluids, tissue homogenates) for the presence of viral antigen.

RE is an electrophoresis of ag into an ab-containing gel. A precipitation line with the shape of a rocket forms. RE is a quantitative technique in as much as the area enclosed by the rocket is directly proportional to the ag/ab ratio of the system. Hyperimmune serum or preferably the immunoglobulin fraction of hyperimmune serum is added to the melted agarose gel.

The amount of serum needed obviously depends on the concentration of precipitating antibody, but it generally varies from 50 - 100 μl for the parvoviruses to 0.5 - 1 ml for the herpesviruses. The agarose used should preferably have a slight EEO eg Litex type HSA. This will sharpen the rockets because the antibodies will be moving slowly in the opposite direction to the antigen.

We use RE as a routine test for the detection of mink enteritis virus in faecal samples. We are at present comparing it with the ELISA test, and it seems that the latter is more sensitive. But taken as a herd test RE seems to be equally well suitable, when representative faecal samples are investigated. RE has the advantage of being easy to read and false positives are almost never seen.

In the laboratory the method is useful for standardizing all sorts of antigens. In addition to mink enteritis virus we use it for other parvoviruses, Aujeszky virus, hog cholera, bovine viral diarrhoea virus (BVDV), for checking foetal calf serum for possible content of antibodies to BVDV,

192

and for screening aborted foetuses for possible content of immunoglobulins (Dalsgaard et al., 1979).

CROSSED IMMUNOELECTROPHORESIS (CIE)

CIE is also an electrophoresis of ag into an ab containing gel, but after the ag mixture has been separated by a primary electrophoresis. The separation step is performed in a non-antibody containing gel (10 V/cm for 2.5 h, agarose type HSA) and a strip of gel (2 x 10 cm) containing the separated substances is transferred to a new plate. Ab containing gel is cast adjacent to the strip, the ag's are electrophoresed into the ab gel, and precipitation arcs are formed (1.5 V/cm overnight, agarose type HSA). The main application of the technique is in the characterization of complex antigenic mixtures, and examples of the identification of more than 30 antigens on one plate have been published (Axelsen et al., 1973).

In virus diagnosis the method has a potential in being a tool for the production of specific antisera to viral antigens. The method is based on the good resolving capacity of CIE. Individual precipitation arcs or normally parts of these can often be cut out of the unstained gel without contamination from other precipitates. The isolated precipitates contain ag, ab, and agarose. If this material is injected into an animal of the same species from which the ab originated, the animal elicits an immune response to the ag only, because the ab is homologous, and the agarose is not immunogenic.

In practice a sufficient quantity of specific antisera can be obtained on average after 3 injections with 2 week intervals. The amount of precipitate needed varies from antigen to antigen. In guinea pigs, rabbits, and pigs we have found that cut material from 2 - 10 CIE plates per injection has been adequate. The agarose pieces are transferred to a syringe, a little buffer is added and the material is homogenized by squeezing it through as fine a needle as possible. An equal part of Freund's incomplete adjuvant is added, and after emulsification it is ready for injection. Using viral antigens it is not always possible to find the precipitates in the unstained gels. We therefore use the procedure to stain one gel, and superimpose the others on the stained gel to locate the precipitates. Naturally it requires strictly standardized conditions to get the precipitate you want in exactly the same position on all the plates. But if following the procedures described above, it is

possible. Certainly, you do not obtain precipitating antisera to all antigens by this method. The precipitates may for unknown reasons be denatured,
poor immunogens etc., but we have found that you have a fairly good chance
that the system works with viral antigens. We have obtained antisera to
ag's from African swine fever virus (Dalsgaard et al., 1977), hog cholera
virus (Dalsgaard Overby, 1977), bovine viral diarrhoea virus, and Aujeszky
virus (Dalsgaard, 1982). The sera are "mono"-specific in as much as they
only produce one precipitation line in CIE. But it has been shown in the
case of glycoproteins from herpes hominis virus that one such line may
contain a complex of a few glycoproteins when subjected to SDS-polyacrylamide gel electrophoresis (Norrild and Vestergaard, 1977). However, the
antisera are normally excellent for diagnostic purposes.

REFERENCES

Axelsen, N.H., Krøll, J. and Weeke, B. 1973. A manual of quantitative
    immunoelectrophoresis. (Blackwell Scientific Publications, Oxford).
Cho, H.J. and Ingram, D.G. 1972. Antigen and antibody in Aleutian
    Disease in mink. 1. Precipitation reaction by agar-gel electrophor-
    esis. J. Immunol., 108, 2, 555-557.
Crowle, A.J. and Cline, L. Jewell. 1977. An improved stain for immuno-
    diffusion tests. J. Immunol. Methods, 17, 379-381.
Dalsgaard, K. 1982. Precipitating antigens involved in protection against
    Aujeszky's disease after natural infection and after immunisation with
    inactivated vaccine. In "Current Topics in Veterinary Medicine and
    Animal Science. Vol. 17" (Eds. G. Wittmann and S.A. Hall) (Martinus,
    Nijhoff, The Hague). pp 107-115.
Dalsgaard, K. and Overby, E. 1977. Immunity against challenge with swine
    fever virus induced by a virus-specified glycopeptide isolated from
    infected cells. In "Agricultural Research Seminar on Hog cholera and
    African swine fever. Hannover, 1977" (CEC publication EUR. 5904)
    (CEC, Luxembourg).pp 70-74.
Dalsgaard, K., Overby, E. and Sanchez-Botija, C. 1977. Crossed immuno-
    electrophoretic characterization of virus-specified antigens in cells
    infected with African swine fever virus. J. Gen. Virol., 36, 203-206.
Dalsgaard, K., Overby, E., Metzger, J.J. and Basse, A. 1979. Rapid
    method for screening of immunoglobulins in porcine fetuses, using
    rocket immunoelectrophoresis. Acta Vet. Scand., 20, 313-320.
Grabar, P. and Williams, C.A. 1953. Methode permettant l'etude conjugee
    des proprietes electrophoretiques d'un melange de proteines; appli-
    cation au serum sanguin. Biochim. biophys. Acta, 10, 193-198.
Norrild, B. and Vestergaard, B.F. 1977. Polyacrylamide gel electrophor-
    etic analysis of herpes simplex virus type 1 immunoprecipitates ob-
    tained by quantitative immunoelectrophoresis in antibody containing
    agarose gel. J. Virol., 22, 113-117.
Pan, I.C., DeBoer, C.J. and Hess, W.R. 1972. African swine fever. Appli-
    cation of immunoelectroosmophoresis for the detection of the antibody.
    Can. J. Comp. Med., 36, 309-316.
Sørensen, K.J. 1980. A serological survey for swine vesicular disease in
    Denmark. Acta Vet. Scand., 21, 324-329.

Sørensen, K.J., Askaa, J. and Dalsgaard, K. 1980. Assay for antibody in pig fetuses infected with porcine parvovirus. Acta Vet. Scand., 21, 312-317.

Terpstra, C. and van Oirschot, J. 1975. Immunoelectroosmophoresis for detection of antibody against swine fever. Agricultural Research Seminar on diagnosis and epizootiology of classical swine fever. Amsterdam 1975. (CEC publication EUR. 5486). (CEC, Luxembourg). pp 198-199.

DIAGNOSTIC USE OF CNS ANTIBODIES

Kurt Danner

Institut fur Hygiene und Infektionskrankheiten der Tiere,
Justus Liebig-Universitat, Giessen, Federal Republic of Germany

ABSTRACT

Antibodies appear in the CNS either by leakage from serum through an
impaired blood-CNS barrier or after local production during certain infections of the CNS, such as distemper in the dog or measles/SSPE in man.
Locally produced CNS antibodies are different from serum antibodies but can
be demonstrated by the same techniques. They may be taken for routine
diagnosis especially when the aetiological agent is difficult to identify.
Our own experiences with Borna disease in horses, sheep and rabbits are
presented, since its diagnosis intra vitam and post mortem is routinely
based upon demonstration of CNS antibodies. It is suggested that the
method might be applicable to other viral infections of the CNS.

INTRODUCTION

Laboratory diagnosis of infectious diseases is optimally achieved by
the demonstration-of the aetiologic agent or its antigens. Whenever aetiologic diagnosis is impossible or unpracticable, eg on account of unsuitable
material or complicated methods, the demonstration of serum antibodies is
preferred. However, interpretation of serologic results is often difficult,
especially if only one serum sample is available; or if the infection is
locally restricted eg to the intestine, and does not produce serologically
manifest immune reactions.

An exceptionally strict localisation does exist in virus infections of
the central nervous system (CNS). Virus multiplication (or persistence),
immune reactions and pathogenetic consequences occur autonomously. The
diagnostic access to these separated events is difficult and intra vitam
only possible by bioptic measurements or puncture of cerebrospinal fluid
(CSF). Post mortem, generally enough material will be available but the
agents involved are often very difficult to cultivate. In many cases, however, specific antibodies are present in the CNS and enable diagnosis intra
vitam and post mortem (Table 1).

This fact has been recognised for many years (Freund, 1930; Kubes and
Gallis, 1944; Kabat et al., 1950) and concerns virus infections as well as
bacterial or toxic diseases (Schliep and Felgenhauer, 1978; Salmi et al.,
1980).

TABLE 1   Laboratory diagnosis of virus infections of the CNS.

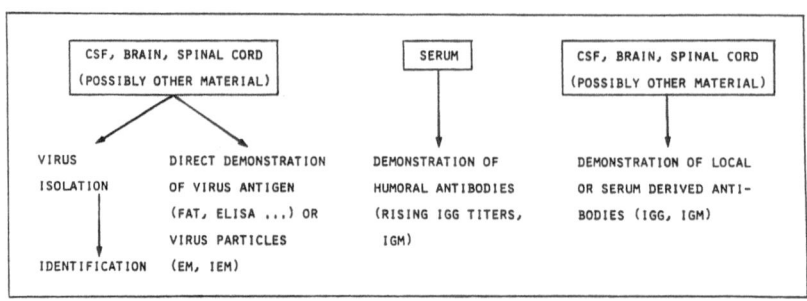

ORIGIN AND FORMATION OF CNS ANTIBODIES

"Humoral" antibodies can be found in the current blood and - in lower
amounts - also in the organs and tissues supplied with blood (blood content;
permeable connection blood-organs). The blood-brain and the blood-CSF barriers, however, impede penetration of substances with molecular weights
higher than 20 000 to 40 000 (Rapoport, 1976; Oehmichen, 1978; Bradbury,
1979) (Fig. 1). Thus, the quantity of antibodies in the CNS remains small
(ratio serum: CSF = 100 - 1 600:1).

Significant amounts of antibodies may be present in the CNS due to
the following events:
1. abnormally high serum levels, eg in cases of multiple myeloma or alco-
    holic cirrhosis of the liver (Schliep and Felgenhauer, 1978);
2. impairment of the blood-CNS barriers; and
3. local formation of antibodies within the CNS.

Although disorders of the blood-CNS barriers may be of diagnostic value
per se, we are more interested in the problems of local antibody formation
in the CNS. Locally produced and mostly secretory antibodies of the IgA
type are relatively well characterised as far as the intestinal tract or
the mammary gland are concerned. In contrast, the immune reactions in the
CNS certainly vary from system to system and are poorly understood in the
individual case.

Local antibody production should be possible:
1. by antigenic stimulation of sessil B-cells in certain regions of the
    brain and spinal cord as well as by lymphocytes within the CSF, or
2. by B-cells (prestimulated ?) migrating from the blood through the intact barriers (a quite astonishing but frequently proven process, cf. Fig. 1).

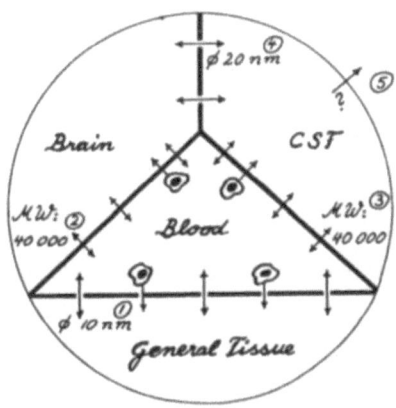

① <u>CONNECTION BLOOD-ORGANS (GENERAL TISSUE)</u>:
   INTERCELLULAR CHANNELS (10 NM WIDTH), PINOCYTOSIS

② <u>BLOOD-BRAIN BARRIER</u>:
   TIGHT INTERCELLULAR JUNCTIONS, NO PINOCYTOSIS,
   TRANSCELLULAR EXCHANGE (CARRIER MEDIATED) UP
   TO MOL. WEIGHT 40,000

③ <u>BLOOD-CSF BARRIER</u>: AS ABOVE

④ <u>BRAIN-CSF BARRIER</u>:
   INTERCELLULAR SPACES (20 NM WIDTH)

⑤ <u>LYMPH DRAINAGE</u> (MECHANISMS UNCLEAR)

Fig. 1   The different compartments of the body.

PROPERTIES OF THE CNS ANTIBODIES

Techniques for the demonstration of CNS antibodies from brain extracts
or CSF correspond to those applied to serum antibodies. Most CNS antibodies described so far (generally in CSF) represent IgG (Salmi et al.,1972;
Vandvik, 1973; Zakay-Rones et al., 1974; Hofmann et al., 1979) although
IgM also occurs (Schliep and Felgenhauer, 1978; Hofmann et al., 1979;
Torrey et al., 1982) and even may be produced over years in the case of
herpes simplex virus encephalitis (Skoldenberg et al., 1981).   In certain
systems eg parainfluenza 6/94 infection in the mouse, IgA predominates over
IgG (Gerhard et al., 1978).

The peculiarities of CNS antibodies (mostly CSF antibodies studied) in
contrast to serum antibodies are their oligoclonal or even monoclonal character (Laterre, 1973) and an enhanced kappa: lambda ratio (Link and

Zettervall, 1970). These characteristics often serve as a diagnostic sign, even without identifying the specificity of the antibodies.

BIOLOGICAL SIGNIFICANCE OF THE CNS ANTIBODIES

There are two mechanisms how antibodies in the CNS may play a role within the pathogenesis of viral diseases:
1. by direct antiviral activity, and
2. by immunepathogenic actions.

The neutralising potency of antibodies in brain or CSF has been proved for some infections, eg canine distemper (Yamanouchi et al., 1979; Tsai et al., 1982), rabies (Bell et al., 1966; Schneider and Burtscher, 1967; Gough et al., 1974), or measles (Brown et al., 1971, 1973; Yamanouchi et al., 1979). In the case of rabies, Bell et al. (1966) frankly consider the presence of antibodies in the brain as a prerequisite for recovery from the disease.

On the other hand, the main pathological event in many infections of the CNS is demyelination (Wisniewski, 1977), which may be due both to a direct cytolytic action of the virus and also to a cytolytic activity of the locally produced antibodies (probably T-cell mediated). One reason for this might be the similarity of viral and cellular antigenic determinants. Examples are the encephalitides due to herpes simplex virus (Russell and Saertre, 1976), to measles/SSPE virus (Oldstone et al., 1975) and to canine distemper virus (Krakowka et al., 1973). Also multiple sclerosis (MS) is a candidate for such mechanisms.

DIAGNOSTIC APPLICATION OF CNS ANTIBODIES

Although the existence of local immune reactions in the CNS has been recognised for many years, their significance for diagnosis has not been widely studied and realised. In the veterinary field, only Borna disease is routinely diagnosed by means of CNS antibodies. Whereas Gough et al. (1974) did not find specific antibodies in the brains of animals which died of rabies, those antibodies are able to differentiate between vaccinated and recovered individuals (Bell et al., 1966) or between postvaccinal encephalitis and recovery (Bell and Moore, 1979). Other work with animals has been carried out under the pathogenetic and comparative point of view. Table 2 summarises some of the studies on CNS antibodies in animals.

In the human field, besides pathogenetic research some diagnostic

TABLE 2   Demonstration of CNS antibodies in animals.

VIRUS/DISEASE	SPECIES	MATERIAL	AUTHORS
EQ. ENCEPHAL.	HORSE	BRAIN	SCHLESINGER, 1949
LOUPING ILL	SHEEP	CSF	REID ET AL., 1971
NEWCASTLE DIS.	CHICKEN	BRAIN	ZAKAY-RONES ET AL., 1974
BORNA DISEASE	VARIOUS	BR.,CSF	DANNER, 1976
CAN.DISTEMPER	MONKEY	CSF	YAMANOUCHI ET AL., 1979
	DOG	CSF	TSAI ET AL., 1982
RABIES	MOUSE	BRAIN, SP.CORD	BELL ET AL., 1966 / GOUGH ET AL., 1974
	DOG	BRAIN	GOUGH ET AL., 1974
	CHICKEN	BRAIN	SCHNEIDER AND BURTSCHER,1967
	GUINEA-PIG	BRAIN, SP.CORD	BELL AND MOORE, 1979 / GOUGH ET AL., 1974
POLIOMYEL.	MONKEY	BRAIN CSF	MORGAN, 1947 / OGRA ET AL., 1973
PARAINFL. 1 (6/94)	MOUSE	CSF	GERHARD ET AL., 1978
MEASLES	MONKEY	CSF	YAMANOUCHI ET AL., 1979

applications have been published (mainly with CSF antibodies). Examples
are given in Table 3. Many efforts have been directed towards the eluc-
idation of the aetiology of MS. A series of viruses have been incriminated
as candidates by the fact that corresponding antibodies could be found in
the CSF of MS patients (eg, measles virus, rubella virus, vaccinia virus
etc.). Until present, however, none of these virus species have been shown
to be responsible for this disease (Arnadottir et al., 1982).

CNS ANTIBODIES IN BORNA DISEASE

As early as 1929, "virulicide" antibodies in the brains of Borna virus
infected rabbits were reported by Nicolau et al. - a statement we were not
able to confirm. But intensive studies into Borna disease were only enabled after we found in vitro methods for the multiplication and identification of Borna virus (Mayr and Danner, 1972, 1974; for a review on Borna
virus and Borna infection see Danner, 1982). Since then, also CNS antibodies have been considered in a scientific as well as a practical sense
(Table 4). In spite of the immense interest in the role which local immune
reactions play within the pathogenesis of Borna infections, CNS antibodies
for us were primarily important - and the only way - for establishing a
routine laboratory diagnosis of this disease, especially in horses

TABLE 3   Demonstration of CNS antibodies in man.

DISEASE/VIRUS	MATERIAL	AUTHORS
ECHO 6	CSF	OGRA, 1970
RSV	CSF	CAPPEL ET AL., 1975
TBE	CSF	HOFMANN ET AL., 1979
JAP. ENCEPH.	CSF	BURKE ET AL., 1982
LCM	CSF	DEIBEL AND SCHRYVER, 1976
HERPES SIMPL.	CSF	RUSSELL AND SAERTRE, 1976 DEIBEL AND SCHRYVER, 1976
MUMPS	CSF	DEIBEL AND SCHRYVER, 1976 NORDAL ET AL., 1978
MEASLES	CSF	DEIBEL AND SCHRYVER, 1976
SSPE/MEASLES	CSF	SALMI ET AL.,1972; NORRBY ET AL., 1973; OLDSTONE ET AL., 1975
	CSF,BRAIN	VANDVIK, 1973
MS/MEASLES	CSF	BROWN ET AL., 1971, 1973 SALMI, 1973; SALMI ET AL., 1972 NORRBY ET AL., 1973 ARNADOTTIR ET AL., 1982
" /VACCINIA	CSF	KEMPE ET AL., 1973 SALMI, 1973; HAIRE, 1976
" /RUBELLA	CSF	SALMI, 1973; HAIRE, 1976 LEBON ET AL., 1976 ARNADOTTIR ET AL., 1982
" /HERPES SIM.	CSF	HAIRE, 1976 ARNADOTTIR ET AL., 1982
" /PARAINFL.2 INFL.A,B, RSV ADENO, MUMPS	CSF	ARNADOTTIR ET AL., 1982
SCHIZOPHRENIA/CMV	CSF	TORREY ET AL., 1982

(Danner, 1976). Indeed, horses infected with Borna virus generally produce only poor serum antibodies or none at all, and virus cultivation from brain material of animals which have died from the disease is often difficult. Fortunately, antibodies regularly occur in the brain and the CSF of infected animals.

For their demonstration, we found the indirect immunofluorescence test (IFAT) specially suited (Danner and Luthgen, 1978). Persistently infected RK 13 cells grown on coverslips and fixed in acetone serve as an antigen substrate. The extraction of brain antibodies is performed by ultra-sonication of a 10% suspension of brain in PBS or tissue culture medium. After centrifugation (15 min at 1,600 g) the supernatant is examined like serum (corresponding brain 1:10). In contrast to many serum samples, brain

TABLE 4   Demonstration of CNS antibodies to Borna disease virus.

ANIMAL	MATERIAL	TECHNIQUE	REMARKS	AUTHORS
RABBIT	BRAIN	NEUTRALIZATION IN VIVO		NICOLAU ET AL., 1929
	BRAIN, CSF, VITREOUS BODY	IFAT, ID, CF	NATURAL AND EXP. INFECTION (I.CER.) MAINLY IGG	DANNER, 1976, 1982 DANNER AND LÜTHGEN, 1978 LÜTHGEN, 1977; METZLER, 1977 LUDWIG ET AL., 1977 METZLER ET AL., 1978
SHEEP	BRAIN, CSF	IFAT	NATURAL INFECTION	DANNER, 1976; METZLER, 1977 METZLER ET AL., 1976, 1979 DANNER AND LÜTHGEN, 1978
HORSE	BRAIN, CSF	IFAT, ID, CF, IMM.ELECTROPH.	NATURAL INFECTION OLIGOCLONAL IGG	DANNER, 1976; METZLER, 1977 LUDWIG AND THEIN, 1977 DANNER AND LÜTHGEN, 1978

material does not lead to nonspecific background staining of the cell cultures.   CSF can be examined undiluted.

TABLE 5   Diagnosis of Borna disease in horses.

HORSE	CLINICAL SUSPICION	EXITUS	ANTIBODIES (IFAT) IN			INF.VIRUS IN BRAIN	ANTIGEN IN BRAIN	HISTOLOGY
			SERUM	CSF	BRAIN			
1:M 9Y	+	EUTH.	1:10	N.D.	1:2560	$10^{3.4}$	N.D.	+
2:M 4Y	+	"	1:20	1:20	1:640	$10^{4.5}$	N.D.	+
5:F ? [*]	?	"	1:40	N.D.	1:10	NEG.	N.D.	+
7:M 6Y	?	"	1:20	1:4	1:40	$10^{4.7}$	+(FAT)	+
9:M 7Y	+	"	1:640	1:160	1:640	$10^{2.4}$	+(FAT)	+
16:F 7Y	+	"	NEG.	1:40	1:40	N.D.	N.D.	+
18:F 20Y	+	DEAD	N.D.	N.D.	1:40	NEG.	+(FAT) 1:640(CF)	+
19:M 3Y	+	EUTH.	1:40	NEG.	1:20	$10^{3.1}$	+(FAT)	+
480:M 12Y	+	"	1:20	1:160	N.D.	N.D.	N.D.	+

[*] : VACCINATION STATUS UNCLEAR

Table 5 shows the diagnostic results in some cases of Borna disease in horses. In all of them, CNS antibodies could be demonstrated, and the disease could always be verified by virus isolation and/or typical histology of the brain. Today, with suspect animals or necropsy material our Borna diagnosis is based exclusively upon the demonstration of antibodies in CSF and/or brain material.

CNS antibodies can also be found in Borna virus infected sheep and rabbits. The quantitative conditions and probably all the immunological events differ between the various species (Table 6). Normally, brain

TABLE 6 Maximal antibody titres (ind. FAT) in Borna virus infected animals.

	SERUM	CSF	BRAIN
HORSE	1:160	1:640	1:1280
SHEEP	1:320	1:80	1:1280
RABBIT	1:20480	1:5120	1:20480

material contains more antibodies than CSF or serum. We were able to follow the infection in sheep, where amounts of antibody found in the serum exceeded that in CSF until about 14 to 18 months after onset of clinical illness, when both titres equalled (Metzler et al., 1979).

Formation and kinetics of brain antibodies were studied in the rabbit after intracerebral infection (Fig. 2). Antibodies first appear in the serum, thus proving that the inoculum also encountered the general tissue and the central immunogenic organs. The CNS antibodies, appearing one week later, are obviously locally produced and not serum derived, since they show extremely high titres and an oligoclonal character (Ludwig et al., 1977). This holds also for naturally infected horses (Ludwig and Thein, 1977). Since immigration of plasma cells into the brain is typical for Borna infections (Anzil and Blinzinger, 1972), those cells might be

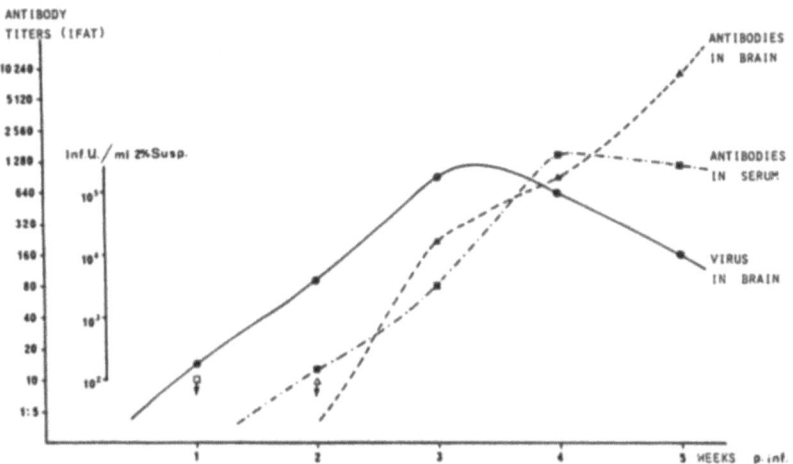

Fig. 2   Production of virus and antibodies in Borna virus infected rabbits (I.Cer.)

responsible for the local antibody production. The chromatographic behaviour of the brain antibodies clearly shows that they mainly belong to the IgG class (Fig. 3, Danner and Luthgen, 1978).

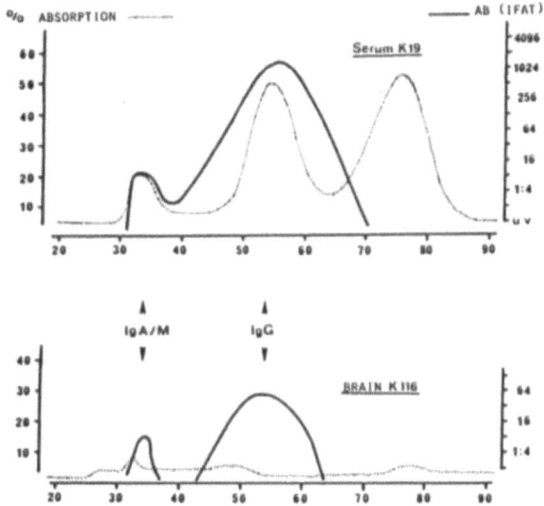

Fig. 3   Chromatographic behaviour of Borna virus antibodies from serum and brain of experimentally infected rabbits (I. Cer.).

For practical purposes, it is important to know that amount of infectivity and antibody content of the brain are reciprocally proportional in early and in late stages of the disease (Fig. 4). In consequences, antibody negative preparations should be tested for infectious virus and vice versa.

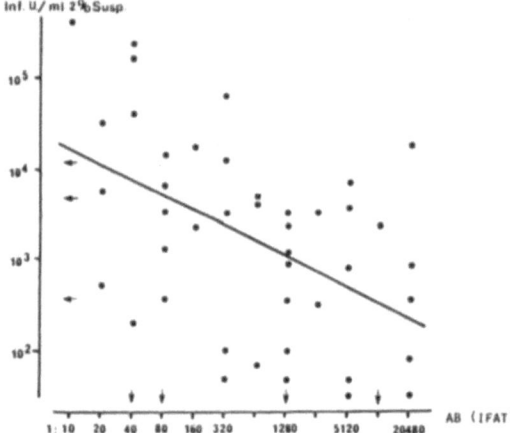

Fig. 4   Ratio virus infectivity: antibodies in the brain of Borna virus infected rabbits (I. Cer.)

An accidental finding was the high antibody content in the vitreous body of experimentally infected rabbits (Fig. 5). The source of these

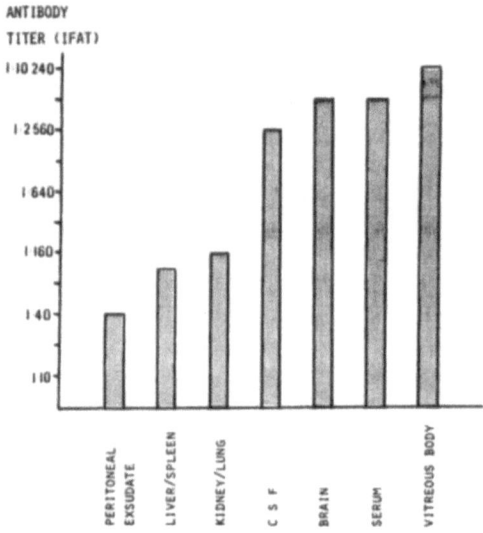

Fig. 5   Antibody content in different substrates of Borna virus infected rabbits (I. Cer.)

antibodies might be the serum, and a low turnover rate of the vitreous tissue would explain the high titres as mere enrichment. On the other hand, why should the antibodies not be produced locally by B-cells present in the

fundus of the eye, a part of the CNS that is notoriously involved in the
pathogenesis of Borna disease (Bemmann, 1926; Krey et al., 1979)?

POSSIBLE APPLICATION IN OTHER INFECTIONS

Before the demonstration of CNS antibodies can be applied to other
infections, one needs to clarify in each system whether the blood-CNS barriers remain intact or not. Antibodies found in the CNS do not always
prove the disease. As a rule however, in normal brain antibodies are not
detectable by routine laboratory techniques. This was shown in our laboratory in a series of brain extracts of various species, where none of
the antibodies usually present in the serum could be detected (eg antibodies to herpesvirus type 1 in the horse, BVD virus in cattle, adenovirus type 1 in dogs, rhinotracheitis and calici viruses in cats etc.). A
significant blood contamination can be eliminated by exsanguinating the
animal prior to removal of the brain (Beam and Allen, 1977).

One must, however, keep in mind that during fetal development the
blood-brain barrier is not established until birth or even later in certain
species (Bradbury, 1979). Thus, in newborn animals maternal antibodies
might appear in the CNS and confuse diagnosis. Indeed, we found antibodies
to canine adenovirus type 1 (contagious hepatitis virus) in the brains of
young puppies. But this fact can be overlooked since infections of the
CNS pose a more serious problem to older individuals.

In a technical respect, one should remember that CSF is differently
composed in the various regions of the body, probably due to the steady
efflux and a short turnover rate. Thus, CSF taken by lumbar puncture contains significantly more antibodies than ventricular CSF (Weisner, 1980).
Species specific differences in formation and circulation of CSF have been
described (Cserr, 1971). Also different regions of the brain may differ in
their antibody content (Mattson et al., 1980).

Finally it has also to be kept in mind that interferon may be produced
in the CNS during some infections, eg canine distemper (Tsai et al., 1982).
Furthermore, substances seem to appear in normal serum and CSF that are
neither antibody nor interferon but inhibit (neutralise?) certain viruses,
eg visna virus (Thormar et al., 1979).

Currently the diagnosis of virus diseases via the demonstration of CNS
antibodies is confined to few infections. Borna disease by chance meets
with all of the indicatory factors shown in Table 7. This will not hold

206

TABLE 7   Arguments pro and contra diagnosis via CNS antibodies.

PRO	CONTRA
SUBACUTE OR CHRONIC DISEASES OR CLINICALLY INAPPARENT INFECTIONS OF THE CNS	PERACUTE DISEASE OF THE CNS (E.G. AUJESZKY'S DISEASE IN DOGS)
DEMONSTRATION OF INFECTIVITY OR VIRAL ANTIGEN IS DIFFICULT (E.G. LATENCY, NO IN VITRO METHOD AVAILABLE ...)	EASY VIRUS IDENTIFICATION
MATERIAL AUTOLYZED	FRESH MATERIAL AVAILABLE
NO SEROLOGICAL MANIFESTATION OF THE INFECTION (E.G. BORNA IN HORSES)	REGULAR FORMATION OF SERUM ANTIBODIES
NO SERUM AVAILABLE (E.G. POST MORTEM)	SERUM AVAILABLE
VACCINATED INDIVIDUALS (CONFUSING SERUM TITERS)	NEWBORN INDIVIDUALS (BLOOD-CNS BARRIER UNDEVELOPED (?))

true for other diseases, but this paper should stimulate further attempts regarding infections like herpesvirus encephalitides in dogs, cats, cattle and horses, tick borne encephalitis in various species, or visna in sheep. On the other hand, in some diseases a lot of conditions will exist that may impede the CNS antibody method. As only one example I should mention Aujeszky's disease in carnivores, where lethal pathogenetic events occur too rapidly to allow formation of antibodies at all.

For all those who understood the title of this paper in another sense, I should add that intracerebral or intrathecal inoculation might be a simple means for the production of highly efficient and monospecific antibody preparations to be used in virologic and diagnostic work.

ACKNOWLEDGEMENTS

Part of the experimental work was done in the Institute of Medical Microbiology, Infectious and Epidemic Diseases, Veterinary Faculty of the University of Munich. The skilled technical assistance of Birgit von Restorff (Munich) and Karin Sacher and Peter Zerche (Giessen) is gratefully acknowledged.

REFERENCES

Anzil, A.P. and Blinzinger, K. 1972. Electron microscopic studies of rabbit central and peripheral nervous system in experimental Borna disease. Acta neuropathol., 22, 305-318.

Arnadottir, T., Reunanen, M. and Salmi, A. 1982. Intrathecal synthesis of virus antibodies in multiple sclerosis patients. Infect. Immun., 38, 399-407.

Beam, T.R. and Allen, J.C. 1977. Blood, brain and cerebrospinal fluid concentrations of several antibiotics in rabbits with intact and inflamed meninges. Antimicrob. Agents Chemother., 12, 710-716.

Bell, J.F. and Moore, G.J. 1979. Allergic encephalitis, rabies antibodies, and the blood/brain barrier. J. Lab. Clin. Med., 94, 5-11.

Bell, J.F., Lodmell, D.L., Moore, G.J. and Raymond, G.H. 1966. Brain neutralization of rabies virus to distinguish recovered animals from previously vaccinated animals. J. Immunol., 97, 747-753.

Bemmann, H. 1926. Beitrag zur pathologischen Histologie, postmortalen Diagnose und Pathogenese der seuchenhaften Gehirn-Ruckenmarksentzundung (Bornasche Krankheit) der Pferde. Vet. Med. Dissertation, Giessen.

Bradbury, M. 1979. Why a blood-brain barrier? Trends NeuroSci., 2, 36-38.

Brown, P., Cathala, F., Gajdusek, D.C. and Gibbs, C.J. 1971. Measles antibodies in the cerebrospinal fluid of patients with multiple sclerosis. Proc. Soc. Exp. Biol. Med., 137, 956-961.

Brown, P., Cathala, F. and Gajdusek, D.C. 1973. Further studies of viral antibodies in the cerebrospinal fluid of patients with multiple sclerosis. Proc. Soc. Exp. Biol. Med., 143, 828-829.

Burke, D.S., Nisalak, A. and Ussery, M.A. 1982. Antibody capture immunoassay detection of Japanese encephalitis virus immunoglobulin M and G antibodies in cerebrospinal fluid. J. Clin. Microbiol., 16, 1034-1042.

Cappel, R., Thiry, L. and Clinet, G. 1975. Viral antibodies in the CSF after acute CNS infections. Arch. Neurol., 32, 629-631.

Cserr, H.F. 1971. Physiology of the choroid plexus. Physiol. Rev., 41, 273-311.

Danner, K. 1976. Labordiagnose der Bornaschen Krankheit uber den Nachweis von Antikorpern im Zentralnervensystem. Zbl. Vet. Med. B., 23, 865-867.

Danner, K. 1982. Borna-Virus and Borna-Infektionen: vom Miasma zum Modell. Enke, Stuttgart.

Danner, K. and Luthgen, K. 1978. Antikorper im ZNS Borna-infizierter Tiere. Fortschr. Vet. Med., 28, 192-197.

Deibel, R. and Schryver, G.D. 1976. Viral antibody in the cerebrospinal fluid of patients with acute central nervous system infections. J. Clin. Microbiol., 3, 397-401.

Freund, J. 1930. Accumulation of antibodies in the central nervous system. J. Exp. Med., 51, 889.

Gerhard, W., Iwasaki, Y. and Koprowski, H. 1978. The central nervous system-associated immune response to parainfluenza type 1 virus in mice. J. Immunol., 120, 1256-1260.

Gough, P.M., Dierks, R.E., Russell, R.M. and Archer, B.G. 1974. Characterisation of brain-associated rabies neutralising substance. J. Infect. Dis., 129, 456-460.

Haire, M. 1977. Significance of virus antibodies in multiple sclerosis. Br. Med. Bull., 33, 40-44.

Hofmann, H., Frisch-Niggemeyer, W., Heinz, F. and Kunz, C.H. 1979. Immuno-

globulins to tick-borne encephalitis in the cerebrospinal fluid of
man. J. Med. Virol., 4, 241-245.
Kabat, E.A., Freedman, D.A., Murray, J.P. and Knaub, V. 1950. A study of
the cristalline albumin, gamma globulin and total protein in the cerebrospinal fluid of one hundred cases of multiple sclerosis. Am. J.
Med. Sci., 219, 55.
Kempe, C.H., Takabayashi, K., Miyamoto, H., McIntosh, K., Tourtellotte, W.W.
and Adams, J.M. 1973. Elevated cerebrospinal fluid vaccinia antibodies in multiple sclerosis. Arch. Neurol., 28, 278-279.
Krakowka, S., McCullough, B., Koestner, A. and Olson, R. 1973. Myelin-
specific autoantibodies associated with central nervous system demyelination in canine distemper virus infection. Infect. Immunol., 8,
819-827.
Krey, H.F., Ludwig, H. and Boschek, C.B. 1979. Multifocal retinopathy in
Borna disease virus infected rabbits. Amer. J. Ophthalmol., 87,
157-164.
Kubes, V. and Gallis, F. 1944. Brain tissue neutralisation, a new biologi-
cal reaction for rabies virus. Can. J. Comp. Med., 8, 48-60.
Laterre, E.C. 1974. Cerebrospinal fluid in pathology. La Ricerca Clin.
Lab., 4, 540-566.
Lebon, P., Schuller, E., Marteau, R. and Lhermitte, F. 1976. Intrathecal
rubella-antibody synthesis in multiple sclerosis. Lancet 1, 689-690.
Link, H. and Zettervall, O. 1970. Multiple sclerosis: disturbed kappa:
lambda light chain ratio of immunoglobulin G in cerebrospinal fluid.
Clin. Exp. Immunol., 6, 435-438.
Ludwig, H. and Thein, P. 1977. Demonstration of specific antibodies in the
central nervous system of horses naturally infected with Borna disease.
Med. Microbiol. Immunol., 163, 215-226.
Ludwig, H., Koester, V., Pauli, G. and Rott, R. 1977. The cerebrospinal
fluid of rabbits infected with Borna disease virus. Arch. Virol., 55,
209-223.
Luthgen, K. 1977. Untersuchungen uber Nachweis, Bildung und Vorkommen von
Bornavirus-Antikorpern. Vet. Med. Dissertation, Munchen.
Mattson, D.H., Roos, R.P. and Arnason, B.G.W. 1980. Isoelectric focusing
of IgG eluted from multiple sclerosis and subacute sclerosing pan-
encephalitis brains. Nature, 287, 335-337.
Mayr, A. and Danner, K. 1972. Production of Borna virus in tissue culture.
Proc. Soc. Exp. Biol. Med., 140, 511-515.
Mayr, A. and Danner, K. 1974. Zuchtung und Titrierung von Borna-Virus in
Zellkulturen aus Organen fotaler Lammer. Zbl. Vet. Med. B., 21,
131-137.
Metzler,A. 1977. Die Diagnose der naturlichen Bornavirus-Infektion bei
Schafen und Pferden. Ein Vergleich verschiedener Methoden. Vet. Med.
Dissertation, Zurich.
Metzler, A., Frei, U. and Danner, K. 1976. Virologisch gesicherter Aus-
bruch der Bornaschen Krankheit in einer Schafherde der Schweiz.
Schweiz. Arch. Tierheilk., 118, 483-492.
Metzler, A., Ehrensperger, F. and Wyler, R. 1978. Naturliche Bornavirus-
Infektion beim Kaninchen. Zbl. Vet. Med. B., 25, 161-164.
Metzler, A., Ehrensperger, F. and Danner, K. 1979. Bornavirus-Infektion
bei Schafen: Verlaufsuntersuchungen nach spontaner Infektion, unter
besonderer Berucksichtigung der Antikorperkinetik im Serum und Liquor
cerebrospinalis. Schweiz. Arch. Tierheilk., 121, 37-48.
Morgan, I.A. 1947. The role of antibody in experimental poliomyelitis.
III. Distribution of antibody in and out of the central nervous system
in paralysed monkeys. Am. J. Hyg., 45, 390.

Nicolau, S., Galloway, I.A. and Stroian, N. 1929. L'immunite dans l'en-
cephalomyelite enzootique experimentale. C.R. Soc. Biol. Paris, 100,
607-610.

Nordal, H.J., Vandvik, B. and Norrby, E. 1978. Multiple sclerosis: Local
synthesis of electrophoretically restricted measles, rubella, mumps
and herpes simplex virus antibodies in the central nervous system.
Scand. J. Immunol., 7, 473-479.

Norrby, E., Salmi, A.A., Link, H., Vandvik, B., Olsson, J.-E. and Panelius,
M. 1974. The measles virus antibody response in subacute sclerosing
panencephalitis and multiple sclerosis. In "Slow Virus Diseases"
(Eds. W. Zeman and E.H. Lennette). (Williams and Wilkins Co., Balti-
more). pp. 72-85.

Oehmichen, M. 1978. Mononuclear phagocytes in the central nervous system.
(Springer, Berlin).

Ogra, P.L. 1970. Distribution of echovirus antibody in serum, naso-
pharynx, rectum and spinal fluid after natural infection with echovirus type 6. Infect. Immun., 2, 150-155.

Ogra, P.L., Ogra, S.S., Al-Nakeeb, S. and Coppola, P.R. 1973. Local antibody response to experimental poliovirus infection in the central
nervous system of rhesus monkeys. Infect. Immun., 8, 931-937.

Oldstone, M.B.A., Bokisch, V.A., Dixon, F.J., Barbosa, L.H., Fucillo, D.
and Sever, J.L. 1975. Subacute sclerosing panencephalitis: Destruct-
ion of human brain cells by antibody and complement in an autologous
system. Clin. Immunol. Immunopathol., 4, 52-58.

Rapoport, S.I. 1976. Blood-brain barrier in physiology and medicine.(Raven
Press, New York).

Reid, H.W., Doherty, P.C. and McAuslan, A. 1971. Louping ill encephalomyelitis in the sheep. III. Immunoglobulins in cerebrospinal fluid.
J. Comp. Pathol., 81, 537-543.

Russell, A.S. and Saertre, A. 1976. Antibodies to herpes-simplex virus
in "normal" cerebrospinal fluid. Lancet I, 64-65.

Salmi, A.A. 1973. Virus antibodies in patients with multiple sclerosis.
Ann. Clin. Res., 5, 319-329.

Salmi, A.A., Panelius, M., Halonen, P., Rinne, U.K. and Penttinen, K. 1972.
Measles virus antibody in cerebrospinal fluids from patients with
multiple sclerosis. British Med. J., 1, 477-479.

Salmi, A.A., Viljanen, M. and Rennonen, M. 1981. Intrathecal synthesis of
antibodies to diphtheria and tetanus toxoids in multiple sclerosis
patients. J. Neuroimmunol., 1, 333-341.

Schlesinger, R.W. 1949. The mechanism of active cerebral immunity to equine
encephalomyelitis virus. J. Exp. Med., 89, 507.

Schliep, G. and Felgenhauer, K. 1978. Serum-CSF protein gradients, the
blood-CSF barrier and the local immune response. J. Neurol., 218,
77-96.

Schneider, L.G. and Burtscher, H. 1967. Untersuchungen uber die Pathogenese der Tollwut bei Huhnern nach intracerebraler Infektion. Zbl.
Vet. Med. B., 14, 598-624.

Skoldenberg, B., Kalimo, K., Carlstrom, A., Forsgren, M. and Halonen, P.
1981. Acta Neurol. Scand., 63, 273. (Cited after Torrey et al., 1982).

Thormar, H., Wisniewski, H.M. and Lin, F.H. 1979. Sera and cerebrospinal
fluids from normal uninfected sheep contain a visna virus inhibiting
factor. Nature, 279, 245-246.

Torrey, E.F., Yolken, R.H. and Winfrey, C.J. 1982. Cytomegalovirus antibody in cerebrospinal fluid of schizophrenic patients detected by
enzyme immunoassay. Science, 216, 892-894.

Tsai, S.C., Summers, B.A. and Appel, M.J.G. 1982. Interferon in cerebro-

spinal fluid. A marker for viral persistence in canine distemper encephalomyelitis. Arch. Virol., 72, 257-265.

Vandvik, B. 1973. Immunopathological aspects in the pathogenesis of subacute sclerosing panencephalitis, with special reference to the significance of the immune response in the central nervous system. Ann.
Clin. Res., 5, 308-315.

Weisner, B. 1980. Unterschiede in der Zusammensetzung von ventrikularem
und lumbalem Liquor. Selektive Funktionen an der Blut-Liquor- und
Hirn-Liquor-Schranke. Lab. Med., 4, 75-80.

Wisniewski, H.M. 1977. Immunopathology of demyelination in autoimmune
diseases and virus infections. Br. Med. Bull., 33, 54-59.

Yamanouchi, K., Sato, T.A., Kobune, F. and Shishido, A. 1979. Antibody
responses in the cerebrospinal fluid of cynomolgus monkeys after intracerebral inoculation with paramyxoviruses. Infect. Immun., 23,
185-191.

Zakay-Rones, Z., Spira, G. and Levy, R. 1974. Local antibody formation in
the brain of chickens. Arch. Virusforsch., 45, 290-293.

LIST OF PARTICIPANTS

BELGIUM

Dr. R. DUCATELLE

Rijksuniversiteit-Gent
Pathologie der Huisdieren
Casinoplein 24
B - 9000 Gent.

Dr. D. PORTETELLE

Universite Libre de Bruxelles
Department de Biologie Moleculaire
Rue des Chevaux 67
1640 Rhode-Saint Genese.

DENMARK

Dr. A.G. BOETNER

Department of Veterinary Virology
and Immunology
The Royal Veterinary and
Agricultural University
Bulowsvej 13
DK - 1870 Copenhagen V.

Dr. K. DALSGAARD

State Veterinary Institute for
Virus Research
Lindholm
DK - 4771 Kalvehave.

Dr. A. MEYLING

State Veterinary Serum Laboratory
Bulowsvej 27
DK -1870 Copenhagen V.

FEDERAL REPUBLIC OF GERMANY

Dr. K. DANNER

Institute fur Hygiene und
Infektionskrankheiten der Tiere
Justus-Liebig-Universitat
Frankfurter Strasse 89
D - 6300 Giessen.

Dr. H.J. THIEL

Bundesforschungsantalt fur
Viruskrankheiten der Tiere
Paul-Ehrlich-Strasse 28
D - 7400 Tubingen.

FINLAND

Dr. T.HYYPIA

University of Turku
Virusopin Laitos
Kiinamyllynkatu 13
SF - 20520
Turku 52.

FRANCE

Dr. A. LABARRE

Ecole National Veterinaire D'Alfort
7 Avenue Du General de Gaulle
94704 Maisons - Alfort Cedex.

Dr. D. LEVY

Laboratoire de Virologie et
 Immunologie des Tumeurs
Hopital Cochin U152
27 rue du Faubourg St Jacques
75014 Paris.

GREECE

Dr. D. BROVAS
Dr. P. VERBELIS

Veterinary Institute of Foot and
 Mouth Disease
Aghia Paraskevi Attikis
Athens.

ITALY

Dr. D. RUTILI

Instituto Zooprofilattico
 Sperimentale
Via S Constanza 14
I - 06100 Perugia.

THE NETHERLANDS

Dr. A.L.J. GIELKENS
Dr. D. HOUWERS
Dr. D. VAN ZAANE
Dr. F. WESTENBRINK

Central Veterinary Institute
Virology Department
Houtribweg 39
8221 RA LELYSTAD.

REPUBLIC OF IRELAND

Dr. P. LENIHAN

Department of Agriculture
Veterinary Research Laboratory
Abbotstown
Castleknock
Co Dublin.

UNITED KINGDOM

Dr. J.A. ALMEIDA

Wellcome Research Laboratories
Langley Court
Beckenham
Kent BR3 3BS.

Dr. M. SEVERIA CAMPO

The Beatson Institute for Cancer
 Research
Wolfson Laboratory for Molecular
 Pathology
Garscube Estate
Switchback Road
Bearsden
Glasgow G61 1BD.

Dr. P.S. GARDNER

Central Public Health Laboratory
Division of Microbiological
 Reagents and Quality Control
175 Colindale Avenue
London NW9 5HT.

Dr. A.J. HERRING

Moredun Institute
408 Gilmerton Road
Edinburgh EH17 7JH.

Prof. J.H. SUBAK-SHARPE

University of Glasgow
Institute of Virology
Church Street
Glasgow G11 5JR.

Dr. R.S. TEDDER

Department of Virology
(Microbiology)
The Middlesex Hospital Medical
School
Riding House Street
London W1P 7LD.

Dr. J.B. McFERRAN
Dr. M.S. McNULTY
Dr. D. TODD

Veterinary Research Laboratories
Stormont
Belfast BT4 3SD.

CEC

Mr. J. CONNELL

Commission of the European
Communities
Room 4/47
86 Rue de la Loi
1049 Brussels
Belgium.